Intimate Partner Violence

Rahn Kennedy Bailey
Editor

Intimate Partner Violence

An Evidence-Based Approach

Springer

Editor
Rahn Kennedy Bailey, MD, DFAPA, ACP
Department of Psychiatry
Charles R. Drew University of Medicine and Science
Los Angeles, CA
USA

ISBN 978-3-030-55863-5 ISBN 978-3-030-55864-2 (eBook)
https://doi.org/10.1007/978-3-030-55864-2

This Springer imprint is published by the registered company Springer Nature Switzerland AG
The registered company address is: Gewerbestrasse 11, 6330 Cham, Switzerland

Foreword

Intimate Partner Violence, IPV, also known as Domestic Violence (DV), has been a problem for many centuries, taking its toll on mental, physical, emotional, and social health. Its devastation cuts across race, class, nationality, and geography. For too many years, the issue was a taboo subject that health providers rarely discussed with patients or directly addressed. As a result of social movements across decades, the 1970s brought about greater awareness and the 1994 federal legislation, the Violence Against Women Act (VAWA). The Violence Against Women Act of 1994 (VAWA) was a United States federal law (Title IV, sec. 40,001-40,703 of the Violent Crime Control and Law Enforcement Act, H.R. 3355) signed as Pub.L. 103–322 by President Bill Clinton on September 13, 1994 (codified in part at 42 U.S.C. sections 13701 through 14,040). The Act provided $1.6 billion toward investigation and prosecution of violent crimes against women, imposed automatic and mandatory restitution on those convicted, and allowed civil redress in cases prosecutors chose to leave un-prosecuted. The Act also established the Office on Violence Against Women within the Department of Justice. VAWA represented a giant step forward in the efforts to prevent IPV, specifically calling upon public health and healthcare providers to do more.

Great work has been done across the United States to bring the issue of IPV to the forefront of social consciousness. Despite the strides forward, there remain marginalized individuals such as women of color and those in the LGBTQ community who have had less favorable outcomes when reporting victimization to authorities. There have been steps backwards, as demonstrated in 2018 with the U.S. Department of Justice's Office on Violence against Women limiting the definition of DV to only acts of physical violence.

This important book not only raises awareness to the issue of IPV, it helps us get back on track by understanding that power and control are the central themes of DV. Debilitating fear, even in the absence of physical injury, is violence. IPV is far more expansive than just physical aggression. IPV includes threats, intimidation, stalking, coercive behavior, and physiological abuse. When power and control over a partner is the rule, social isolation often results. Victims are told what to do, where to go, how to spend their money (if they are allowed to have any), and with whom they can interact. Having to live a life under the constant threat of abuse has grave consequences, including debilitating fear. One woman, who served as faculty with me in a violence prevention class at the Harvard School of Public Health, told the story of being overcome with fear and frustration while in a store trying to decide upon which shampoo to buy. At the time, she was a year out of a relationship, clear across country, and living pretty much incognito and on her own for the first time in a couple of months when she realized that she could not make that simple decision without tremendous fear—while in the abusive relationship, every decision she made carried the threat of a violent response from her abuser.

Many victims feel they are to blame for the abuse they endure, a wrong that providers are called to address. Over time, a victim's self-esteem and self-worth can deteriorate. If a victim is reticent and hopeless, they are less likely to disclose abuse to providers. Additionally, consideration must be given to the tremendous fear that a victim may feel of further abuse, often a direct result of in experience. Abusers make overt threats to harm or kill if abuse is ever disclosed. Fear of the next abusive act, endangering their children, loss of financial stability, or even the loss of life are all real barriers that can prevent a victim from seeking help.

Medical professionals play an important role in identifying victims of abuse. Victims of IPV tend to seek medical attention for various problems at rates higher than the general population. Contrary to popular belief, most victims of domestic violence are not battered and bloody when they seek medical attention. Victims have mental health complaints such as anxiety and depression. It is also common for victims to complain of less easily identified gastrointestinal, gynecological, and diffuse pain complaints. It often requires sensitive inquiry for healthcare professionals to identify a victim of abuse. Substance use and abuse are also associated with IPV and can be the presenting symptom. Healthcare professionals are uniquely positioned to talk to victims in a confidential and private setting. Health providers must be properly educated to provide resources, empathy, understanding, and validation to victims.

In addition to physical symptoms, there are emotional/mental health symptoms caused by or associated with IPV that include depression, anxiety, and PTSD. Also, the cycle of abuse, those exposed to victimization becoming perpetrators, is evident in some IPV situations. For example, after preforming valiantly and experiencing the burdens of war, soldiers may return home to become victims or perpetrators of abuse. Another example of this cycle is children who witness IPV are at risk for both psychological and physical harm. Early life exposure may set the "norm" for what is appropriate in a relationship and place a child at risk for become either a victim or perpetrator of violence, including IPV.

Competent trained providers are required to address special populations experiencing IPV. For example, law enforcement couples have an IPV rate that is almost double the national average and in that setting calling the police for protection can become complicated, impractical, and even dangerous when an abuser is a law enforcement officer. Police officers are trained to control others, a skill that can make them dangerous abusers. Additionally, the possession of and ready access to firearms in those magnifies the gravity of physiological and physical suffering a victim must endure. Because of historic cultural and professional bias, women of color and members of the LGBTQ community may also require particular attention.

Homelessness, another significant health risk, can impact IPV. A competent professional is critical in these settings.

Abuse is never acceptable. Cultural differences in how IPV is viewed and understood, notwithstanding providers, must identify and address IPV. Patriarchal societies that emphasize a man's authority and minimize a woman's autonomy may make identifying and addressing IPV difficult. A cultural competent provider can better identify problems and offer realistic, practical responses.

Women are approximately 85% of the victims of IPV. Both men and women can be victimized in heterosexual and same sex relationships. *Breaking the Surface: The Greg Louganis Story* clearly and poignantly describes a same sex abusive relationship with all the dynamics of power and control and fear. In Louganis' situation, financial freedom, which is often protective against abuse, was not a factor. Men are not just the perpetrators of abuse and women are not just victims of abuse. Though their motives may vary, women do abuse their male partners. Similarly, male victims experience shame, guilt, and helplessness. Men express fear that if their abuser is a woman, their complaints will not be taken seriously and they will be labeled as the abuser, despite being the victim. If a celebrity or athlete is involved in IPV as an abuser, it can appear in the national spotlight, often reflecting a message that these individuals can perpetrate acts of domestic violence with impunity, giving an impression of IPV as a consequence-free act.

This book, with its clear call for more effective healthcare providers who completely embrace IPV as their responsibility, set the stage for:

- Better provider protocols and responsiveness to both women and men who experience IPV.
- Strengthening the #MeToo movement.
- Staying the course when it comes to exposing the inequalities and injustices and the social norms that undergird them.
- Increasing the culturally competent outreach and response to women and men victimized by domestic violence who are seeking assistance.

Because of this book, we know more. Because we know more, we must do more.

Deborah Prothrow-Stith, MD
Charles R. Drew University of Medicine and Science, College of Medicine,
Los Angeles, CA, USA

Preface

Domestic violence remains a prevalent issue in American society and impacts individuals from every class, gender, race, culture, and sexual orientation. Over time, the once taboo subject of Intimate Partner Violence (IPV) has evolved into a common conversational topic that is splashed across national headlines. When media attention is brought to the issue of IPV, it is often a celebrity or an athlete who appears in the national spotlight. Unfortunately, many of these individuals perpetrate acts of domestic violence with impunity. Rarely is jail time given. This can create the false image of IPV as a consequence-free act. Both past and future legislation that offers protections and services for victims of abuse aide in working against that notion. However, there are still marginalized individuals such as those in the LGBTQ+ community who have less favorable outcomes when reporting victimization to authorities. Great work has been done to bring the issue of IPV to the forefront of social consciousness. However, even modern official definitions limit the acts that may be considered as IPV. In 2018, the U.S. Department of Justice's Office on Violence Against Women limited the definition of domestic violence to only include acts of physical violence.

Medical professionals play an important role in identifying victims of abuse. Victims of IPV tend to seek medical attention at rates higher than the general population. Contrary to popular belief, most victims of domestic violence are not battered and bloody when they seek medical attention. Victims have mental health complaints such as anxiety and depression. It is also common for victims to complain of less easily identified gastrointestinal, gynecological, and diffuse pain complains. It often requires sensitive inquiry for healthcare professionals to identify a victim of abuse. Healthcare professionals are in a unique position to be able to talk to victims in a confidential and private setting. They must be properly educated to provide resources, empathy, understanding, and validation to victims.

Men are not the only perpetrators and women are not the only victims of abuse. This dynamic is examined in this book. Though their motives may vary, women do abuse their male partners. Similarly, male victims experience shame, guilt, and helplessness. A fear echoed by many men is that their complaints will not be taken seriously. Worse still, some men fear that if authorities were involved, they would still be (and often are) labeled as the abuser. This theme is carried out in non-heterosexual relationships as well. Those in the LGBTQ community experience and inflict abuse as well. Similarly, society's view of perceived power equality in non-heterosexual relationships may make it easy to dismiss IPV in these groups. Reporting IPV to authorities in these groups can be problematic. Often, authorities may make false assumptions as to who is the perpetrator or victim.

This textbook is designed to present a comprehensive update covering the psychopathology and epidemiology of domestic violence, accompanied by related medical and legal considerations. The introductory parts will discuss more general themes such as defining domestic violence, exploring statistics in various populations, and barriers to recognition and reporting. The major body of the book, however, will consist of chapters devoted to individual topics important to understanding domestic violence in various communities and subgroups. These topics will examine many of the dynamics of domestic violence, such as factors associated with victimization, disparities and special populations, subtypes of offenders, unique ethical and legal components of victim, offender evaluations, the impact of gun ownership/accessibility, sexual violence, domestic homicide, and the prevention of repeated offenses. The chapters will include resources and guidelines when available.

This text seeks to navigate this changing landscape by looking at domestic violence from a broader perspective in an attempt to tackle an increasingly underreported and underrecognized problem. Further, the text will explore the psychological, social, and economic burdens of domestic violence as well as the current medical and legal approaches to managing victims and offenders. The book will be a unique contribution to the field. Existing texts focus mainly on domestic violence support and education from field workers and victims along with psychology-based texts that are geared towards professional audiences. By including transdisciplinary perspectives from advocacy resources, public health, forensic psychiatry, and legal sources, this book will provide a practical and useful resource with wide applicability.

The Covid-19 Pandemic started as our team was finishing the details of writing this textbook. As more and more family members were forced to quarantine together, the reports of family/ domestic related violence increased. Fragile and already-stressed relationships were pushed over the "barely functioning" threshold into the realm of violence, both emotionally and physically. Loss of loved ones, employment, financial stability, and simply freedoms we all take for granted catapulted the world into stressful tizzy. At this moment, more than ever before, increasing awareness of Intimate Partner Violence (IPV) is crucial.

Rahn Kennedy Bailey, MD, DFAPA, ACP
Charles R. Drew University of Medicine and Science,
College of Medicine, Kedren Community Health Center,
Los Angeles, CA, USA

Acknowledgements

It takes a great amount of effort to bring a collaboration such as this book to fruition. Many who assisted are not listed as authors but whose efforts have made this publication a reality. To all of them, I am grateful for your steadfast support and contributions. Below are those student researchers and medical trainees whose efforts were seminal:

Mohayed Mohayed, MD—First Year Psychiatry Resident, Charles R. Drew Medical University.
Ebone Bailey—L1 Law Student, Northwestern California University School of Law, and Research Assistant at Bailey Psychiatric Associates.
Kim Arrington, PsyD—Head of Psychology, Garnet Health Medical Center.
Kevin Lemaire, DO, MS—Chief Resident, Garnet Health Medical Center.
Sheena Sharpe, DO, MS—PGY 1 Psychiatry Resident, Garnet Health Medical Center.
Amit Grover, MBBS—Research Associate, Kedren Community Health Center.
Omar Merino—Academic Administrator of Clerkship and Residency.

As I wrote this book addressing Intimate Partner Violence, I was struck by the recent activity around the issue of violence in our society. Violence anywhere can be a threat to safety everywhere. The recent array of violent deaths across our country has focused a spotlight on violent trends against those who are susceptible, marginalized, and vulnerable. Thus, as I reflect on the issue of violence, I am fortunate that in my own life I have benefited by being mentored by several men who safeguarded and defended their families and communities. Two in particular were my father Edward Mitchell Bailey and father-in-law Reney Barlow. I dedicate this book to their loving memory.

Finally, to my brand-new grandson Jeremy Michael Mason Jr., born on June 29, 2020, this is my effort to make this world a safer place for you.

Los Angeles, CA, USA — Rahn Kennedy Bailey, MD, DFAPA, ACP

Contents

Contributors

Rahn Kennedy Bailey, MD, DFAPA, ACP Department of Psychiatry, Charles R. Drew University of Medicine and Science, Los Angeles, CA, USA

Theresa A. Bailey, MA, HS-BCP Bailey Psychiatric Associates, Houston, TX, USA

Janice M. Beal, EdD, MPH Beal Counseling Associates, Houston, TX, USA

Tiffani L. Bell, MD Wake Forest School of Medicine, Department of Child and Adolescent Psychiatry, Winston-Salem, NC, USA

Ludmila De Faria, MD, DFAPA Department of Psychiatry, University of Florida College of Medicine, Gainesville, FL, USA

Dashiel J. Geyen, EdD, MPH Prairie View A & M University, Prairie View, TX, USA

Candace Mason, MD, MS Department of Orthopaedic Surgery, Keck School of Medicine of USC, Los Angeles, CA, USA

Roger A. Mitchell, MD, FASCP, OCME Chief Medical Examiner of the District of Columbia, Washington, DC, USA

Mohayed Mohayed, MD Charles R. Drew University College of Medicine, Los Angeles, CA, USA

Maureen Sayres Van Niel, MD Steering Committee, United States Department of Health and Human Services Women's Preventive Services Initiative, 2016–19, President, American Psychiatric Association Women's Caucus, Chair, Committee of Minority and Underrepresented Groups, American Psychiatric Association, Psychiatrist and Private Consultant, Cambridge, MA, USA

A. Dexter Samuels, PhD, MHA Center for Health Policy, Meharry Medical College, Nashville, TN, USA

Terrence Schofield, PhD, MS Walden University, Minneapolis, MN, USA

Kathy C. Scott-Gurnell, MD, MS Child & Adolescent Psychiatrist, Pearland, TX, USA

Derek H. Suite, MD, MS Teachers College, Columbia University, New York, NY, USA

Conte Terrell, PhD Fresh Spirit Wellness for Women, Inc., Houston, TX, USA

Mark H. Townsend, MD, MS George C Dunn Professor of Psychiatry, Louisiana State University Health Sciences Center New Orleans, New Orleans, LA, USA

Ulrick Vieux, DO, MS Chairman and Psychiatry Residency Program Director at Garnet Health Medical Center, Middletown, NY, USA

Mallory Williams, MD, MPH, FACS, FICS, FCCP, FCCM Howard University Hospital, Washington, DC, USA

Howard University College of Medicine, Washington, DC, USA

Howard University National Center of Excellence for Trauma & Violence Prevention, Washington, DC, USA

Overview of Intimate Partner Violence

1

Maureen Sayres Van Niel

I have spent decades as a physician specializing in women's health and mental health on a national level, but I will never forget my experience as I sat at a meeting in Washington, D.C., one morning a few years ago. I was not surprised by the presenter's first statement that 4 out of 5 victims of intimate partner violence (IPV) are women, but I will never forget the disbelief I felt when he stated that *77% of women in jail in the United States and 80% of homeless women with children are survivors of intimate partner violence.* That can't be true, I challenged. Those figures suggest that IPV is the root cause of a high percentage of the physical, emotional, and financial difficulties that women face in the United States.

Sadly, it *is* true, and since that time I have set my approach to women's health and mental health into a context in which I realize not only the enormous scope of intimate partner violence but also its devastating long-term ramifications in victims' lives—and specifically, the inextricable likely causal relationship between IPV and homelessness, mental and physical health disorders, incarceration, and substance abuse, some of the most severe health and economic problems confronting American women.

The scope of intimate partner violence is staggering: About 24 Americans per minute are victims of rape, physical violence or stalking by an intimate partner, adding up to millions of victims per year. The national support hotline for victims of intimate partner violence receives an average of 20,000 calls per day—an unfathomable number. While much of this book focuses on women as victims, people of all genders can be victims of IPV, and, in addition, disabled individuals are frequent victims of IPV. IPV is a problem whose scope is broad and deep. About 1 out of 4 women and 1 out of 10 men have been the victim of severe physical violence by an

M. S. Van Niel (✉)
Steering Committee, United States Department of Health and Human Services Women's Preventive Services Initiative, 2016–19, President, American Psychiatric Association Women's Caucus, Chair, Committee of Minority and Underrepresented Groups, American Psychiatric Association, Psychiatrist and Private Consultant, Cambridge, MA, USA

R. K. Bailey (ed.), *Intimate Partner Violence*,
https://doi.org/10.1007/978-3-030-55864-2_1

intimate partner in their lifetime. In addition, nearly 1 out of 5 women have been raped in their lifetime. These numbers are decidedly less than the true incidence of IPV, since a high proportion of victims are afraid to report such violence or seek medical help for their injuries for fear of retaliation by the abuser or for fear of discrimination by authorities who may not take their reports seriously.

Think about this with regard to the women in your own life: That's one out of every four of our sisters, mothers, grandmothers, and daughters—one out of four of our female friends, neighbors, teachers, and doctors—who have experienced severe intimate partner violence. IPV knows no boundaries when it comes to income, gender, race, sexual orientation, or age; it is a scourge present in every subgroup of society. IPV is a pervasive problem of overwhelming importance, with implications for the public health of all Americans.

Another important factor to take into account when discussing IPV is that IPV disproportionately affects women of color. To more comprehensively care for IPV victims, it is necessary to consider the sociopolitical factors at play in many victims' lives, and barriers such as racism, mistrust of medical or law enforcement figures, poverty, discrimination, trauma, or immigration status play important roles in the treatment of IPV victims. By taking action to correct these inequities and social determinants, health disparities can be reduced and overall health outcomes improved.

***

Chapter by chapter, this book eloquently describes the evidence-based diverse aspects of intimate partner violence. Some of the things you will learn while reading this book are that Native Americans and Alaskan Natives are currently the racial group with the highest incidence of IPV and that bisexuals are currently the sexual orientation group with the highest incidence of IPV. You will also learn that the use of alcohol or drugs like cocaine and meth markedly increase the incidence of IPV; that occupations with high rates of abusers include extremely stressful, violence-related jobs such as those in the military, law enforcement, and corrections; and that the murder of an intimate partner occurs at the rate of about three people per day in the United States, with guns involved in about half of those murders.

To improve your understanding of what you're about to read, it is important to clarify several terms used in this book:

First, many people are confused by the different terms used to describe abuse. Is *domestic violence* the same thing as *intimate partner violence*? If not, what is the difference?

For decades during the last century, abuse in a personal relationship was characterized as *domestic violence*, a term that implied the standard model of a heteronormative male-female marriage. Over time we have come to realize that violence can in fact occur in any type of intimate relationship: whether the partners are married or unmarried; between partners of any gender, gender identity or sexual orientation, with siblings or other relatives; or in any intimate relationship, such as with a teacher or coach. Consequently, to be more accurate and inclusive, the term *intimate partner violence*, or *IPV*, was coined and that term prevails in the literature today. When IPV occurs in a dating relationship between teenagers, it is called teen dating violence. IPV does not include child abuse, which is a different category defined as the abuse of anyone under the age of 18, no matter who the abuser might be (e.g., a parent, coach, teacher, clergyperson, or another person under the age of 18 whom the victim may or may not be dating).

Second, some people are confused about which behaviors actually constitute intimate partner violence. Is it IPV only if one partner beats or physically harms the other partner? The answer is no. IPV can take several forms: physical, psychological/emotional, sexual, and financial abuse, as well as stalking, cyberstalking, and human trafficking.

- IPV can consist of *physical acts of violence*, such as hitting, strangling, kicking, pushing, biting, burning, suffocating, or physically restraining a person in any way. The presence of a gun in the home dramatically increases the risk of homicide. Abusers are often drinking alcohol to excess or using drugs when the abuse occurs.
- IPV often relies on coercive control and can also take the form of constant *psychological/emotional abuse*, including a pattern of coercion, constant criticizing or berating, and intimidation of an intimate partner. The goal of emotional abusers is often to isolate their victims in order to prevent them from reporting the abuse to relatives or friends. When people experience this form of abuse over time, it has a damaging psychological effect, with victims developing low self-esteem and ultimately, even sometimes feeling that they do not deserve anything better than abusive treatment. Some individuals who have been emotionally abused as children have an especially difficult time escaping the psychological cycle that chronic abuse creates, and without help they are at greater than usual risk for becoming either victims or abusers in their own adult relationships.
- IPV can also take the form of forcing someone to have *unwanted sexual contact*. In fact, sexual assault is a common form of coercion or violence, occurring in just under half of all relationships with IPV—and approximately half of all female rape victims were raped by an intimate partner. The designation of abuse also applies when the victim is unable to give consent to a sexual act, such as if the person is intoxicated or cognitively or physically impaired.
- IPV can also take the form of exerting *financial control* over an intimate partner's life. This type of abuse often consists of threatening to cut off financial support so that the victim cannot leave the home, preventing the victim from accessing family money or refusing to allow the victim to work outside the home. It can also take the form of threatening to harm the victim's child, pet, or property unless the abuser has complete financial control. Many victims lose their jobs because of missed days at work and other consequences of the abuse, producing national as well as personal economic consequences.
- IPV can also consist of *stalking, harassing, or cyberstalking* an intimate partner or former intimate partner, a common problem that has increased in incidence over recent years. The definition of *stalking* includes physically confronting a person at home or work; making unwanted phone, text, IM, or email contact with someone; watching, following, or recording someone with-

out permission; and sending unwanted gifts. Recent technological innovations have allowed this form of IPV to also include cyberstalking or bullying—using social media or the Internet in general to bully, harass, or post revealing private information or photographs of a person without permission. Almost two-thirds of all stalking victims were stalked by an intimate partner or former intimate partner, and many of those murdered by a partner were previously stalked by that person.
- IPV can also consist of *human trafficking*—capturing individuals and forcing them to do labor or sexual acts for the financial gain of their captors, the traffickers. This disturbing and all-too widespread form of abuse often victimizes individuals in vulnerable situations, such as recent immigrants who have been promised high-paying jobs or young people who have run away from home and have nowhere to live. Many victims of human trafficking are tricked or manipulated into captivity by individuals who force them into physical intimacy, either with themselves or clients. These victims are then held against their will, unable to escape.
- IPV can occur between people of all genders. Victims of same-sex IPV may be even less likely to report it, depending on their level of comfort about disclosing their sexual orientation. In fact, those who feel they must keep their sexuality secret may be even more easily controlled by violent partners. Moreover, law enforcement members struggling to identify a victim and perpetrator can be ill prepared to respond to interpersonal violence among non heterosexual partners. They and other responders may not even recognize the nature or severity of the violent acts they witness between same-sex sexual partners, assigning equal blame, rather than identifying a victim and a perpetrator.

The long-term physical and mental health consequences of IPV can be devastating. The physical effects on victims include unwanted pregnancy or complications of pregnancy such as low birth weight, pregnancy loss, and hemorrhage. Victims may become infected with HIV or another sexually transmitted disease or infection and may also experience a higher incidence of early heart disease, asthma, stroke, traumatic brain injury, chronic gastrointestinal and pain conditions, and obesity. The mental health effects include poor self-esteem; higher rates of severe or mild PTSD, anxiety and depressive disorders, somatoform disorders such as malingering, substance use disorders; and higher rates of suicide attempts, completed suicides, and being murdered.

One chapter of this book addresses the fact that adults are not the only victims of IPV. The presence of IPV between adults in the home also has a lasting effect on the growth and development of children in the household because many of them have witnessed the abuse throughout their childhoods. Many parents are concerned about the effects of IPV on their children; these effects can be both short- and long-term mental and physical health problems that vary depending on the age of the child. Children in households where IPV occurs may often also be experiencing their own abuse, at the hand of the same abusers, so they should be carefully monitored for child abuse. Furthermore, as they grow up, children who have witnessed IPV are at risk for repeating IPV behaviors—as either the abuser or the victim—in their own relationships. Interrupting the cycle of abuse with identification and treatment is critical to enabling these children to be physically and emotionally healthy.

There is a direct and overwhelming evidence-based correlation between the experience of adult IPV and a marked increase in physical and mental health problems; incarceration; drug, nicotine, and alcohol addiction; homelessness; early death from suicide and violent death at the hands of the abuser; and severe structural competency problems such as poverty, racism, hunger, job loss, and lack of education. The problem of intimate partner violence, I have come to realize, is at the heart of why so many individuals fail to progress in their lives. It is coercive control that impairs their financial well-being, their physical health, their mental health and self-esteem, their ability to feel safe whether alone or when parenting children, and their ability to achieve what they are capable of in their lifetimes. When we become aware, as we have over the past few decades, of the direct and alarming relationship between being a victim of IPV and all these adverse outcomes, it is imperative that we take action to prevent, diagnose, and treat the problem at its origin. Our failure to do so has already had disastrous consequences.

After you read this informative book, you will see the critical importance of educating all individuals to recognize when they are in an abusive situation, of requiring healthcare providers to ask their patients of all genders if they are experiencing IPV, to be monitoring their children for signs of abuse, to have resources available to those who are experiencing abuse, and to take taking clear and definitive steps to interrupt the deadly IPV that has destroyed so many lives.

Intimate partner violence is always wrong, regardless of the form it takes. Our failure to act to solve the problem of IPV is closely connected to our failure as a society to address serious issues that most often affect women and the most vulnerable members of our society, our children. It is a telling commentary on our societal values that 77% of women in jail and 80% of homeless women with children are abuse survivors—and it should serve as a call to action for all of us to reevaluate our current judicial system's treatment of victims and our tendency as a society to tolerate this level of injustice to victims and their children. Let us protect these victims of intimate partner violence using all the resources we can bring to bear. And let this book begin the effort to address this pervasive and life-threatening problem head on.

And finally, many of you who are reading this book may currently be victims or perpetrators of intimate partner violence. The first step you can take is to ask for help right now from anyone you feel you can trust. You can call a 24-hour National Domestic Violence Hotline, *1-800-799-7233*, and speak anonymously to an understanding person about your situation, who will provide comfort and guidance at any time of the day or night. You can also use the hotline website's online chat feature at the thehotline.org [1]. You are most certainly not alone: You can get help with this problem and take meaningful action to restore your life, no matter how badly it is broken.

Reference

1. National Domestic Violence Hotline. https://www.thehotline.org/

Intimate Partner Violence in the Healthcare Setting

2

Candace Mason

Intimate partner violence (IPV) and its consequences are common healthcare concerns. This chapter will explore the role of the healthcare provider in identifying and aiding victims of IPV.

Incidences of IPV are ubiquitous and cases are reported throughout the world. The impacts of enduring sexual or physical violence at the hands of an intimate partner can cause physical and emotional suffering. Often, victims of abuse will seek medical aid for their many and varied symptoms. Particular attention must be taken by healthcare providers to investigate the cause of a suspected victim's symptoms. This chapter will describe some common physical and behavioral clues exhibited by victims of IPV. It is the informed healthcare provider who may be able to constellate the signs and symptoms that may appear mystifying when viewed in isolation.

Intimate partner violence is a common phenomenon, with about 15–71% of women reporting having experienced IPV over their lifetime [1]. Additionally, it is important to know that victims of abuse seek medical attention at rates higher than their non-abused counterparts, accounting for them being three times more likely to seek treatment at an emergency room [2]. As will be discussed throughout this book, there is a common theme that the abusive partner is often controlling and domineering. The perpetrator of abuse typically keeps the victim of abuse socially isolated. Any medical exam or consultation may be one of the few times a victim of abuse is not under the controlling and watchful eye of their abuser. This puts the healthcare provider in a unique position to both investigate and address intimate partner violence.

Typically, the idea of intimate partner violence conjures up the image of a battered woman seeking acute treatment for her physical injuries in an emergency room setting. Though these scenarios certainly happen, the aim of this chapter is to

C. Mason (✉)
Department of Orthopaedic Surgery, Keck School of Medicine of USC,
Los Angeles, CA, USA

R. K. Bailey (ed.), *Intimate Partner Violence*,
https://doi.org/10.1007/978-3-030-55864-2_2

highlight the fact that a healthcare provider is much more likely to see a victim of intimate partner abuse during routine medical exams or follow-ups. It is during these subtler and routine presentations that a care provider is provided with a golden opportunity to provide aid and insight to prevent a future overt presentation and consequence of abuse such as severe trauma, sudden homelessness, or death (a crisis).

Victims of intimate partner violence experience a myriad of concomitant health issues. Victims of IPV have more self-reported gastrointestinal complaints. These symptoms can range in severity from loss of appetite to eating disorders and stress-associated irritable bowel syndrome. A very common complaint in women who experience intimate partner violence is gynecological symptoms.

Symptoms may include pain during intercourse, decreased sexual desire, vaginal bleeding, pelvic pain, and urinary tract infections (UTIs). These symptoms likely arise from undesired sexual intercourse and the associated physical trauma. Furthermore, the abusive partner may refuse to use protection or birth control methods; this may lead to sexually transmitted infection and unintended pregnancy. Women who experience intimate partner violence are twice as likely to be hospitalized during the antenatal period. These hospitalizations were not associated with delivery [1].

An astute healthcare provider should consider the possibility of IPV when confronted with a patient with atypical or otherwise unaccounted for pain or dysfunction. Similarly, women who have suffered acute physical violence and are seen in a healthcare setting tend to present with a similar pattern of injuries. Annually, 40–60% of women in a violent relationship sustain injuries to the face, neck, and chest [3].

One missed bruise may be a missed opportunity to uncover abuse.

Paying consideration to above, a healthcare provider may observe a pattern of behavior and clinical signs that may suggest IPV. A victim may request to be seen on multiple visits and report only vague complaints. A woman may have a past medical history of repeat miscarriages, terminated pregnancies, or pre-term labor. If an injury is investigated, the victim may downplay the seriousness or give an inconsistent reason as to how the injury was sustained. If a victim is seen in a healthcare setting with their partner, a provider should be mindful to note if the partner is aggressive or speaks for the patient. This, along with observable hesitation or fear to speak while the partner is present, can be signs of abuse. Depression and anxiety are other common presenting symptoms of those suffering from intimate partner abuse. A victim may be noncompliant with medication if they feel that the underlying causes of their symptoms were not addressed.

Healthcare providers are familiar with mental health problems from which patients may suffer. In particular, many patients wrestle with anxiety and depression. Interestingly, unipolar depressive disorders are the second leading cause of disease burden in women aged 15–44 years old worldwide [4]. Equipped with this knowledge, healthcare providers should be cognizant of the association between IPV victimization and depression. It is easy to imagine how the trauma of violence, the menace of future violence, and an unhappy/dysfunctional intimate relationship can lead to depression. However, there are some other initially confounding patterns noticed when regarding mental health and IPV. Some have suggested that depression and other mental health maladies may precipitate IPV victimization [4]. Studies among US teenagers suggest that depression precedes first incidents of dating violence [4] (see Chap. 14).

At a glance, this seems as though IPV and depression are inexorably linked and self-perpetuate each other. However, due to depressed states, teenagers are less selective in their choosing or acceptance of a partner. Thus, depressed teens couple with an individual who has poor impulse control or is susceptible to violence [4]. In either case, a depressed patient may be quietly suffering from or at high risk for future IPV. Again, a patient who is diagnosed with depression, on antidepressants, or complaining of depressive symptoms may be experiencing IPV victimization. Good clinical judgment and a genuine concern for the patient's health and safety should guide a provider to explore the nature/quality of the patient's relationship with their partner and the possibility of intimate partner violence.

Indeed, there are mental health consequences for those suffering from abuse. Many victims may report anxiety, depression, or PTSD. Naturally, one would expect living with the constant prospect of physical violence and the associated psychological disorder to be burdensome. Some victims of abuse turn to substance use to help cope with the difficulties of an abusive intimate relationship. It is observed that substance use within a relationship may increase the likelihood of violence. Forty to sixty percent of married or cohabiting patients entering treatment for substance abuse reported one or more episodes of partner violence in the year prior to program entry [5].

The reasons why intimate partner violence occurs are various and complex. Likely, it involves social, psychological, environmental, and contextual factors. Substance use in itself has not been identified as a causative factor for IPV perpetration or victimization, although there is a consensus that those who engage IPV often drink alcohol or use drugs [5]. Intoxication often accompanies violence [5]. Here are some alarming statistics relating to IPV and substance use (particularly alcohol). Over half of IPV victims state that their abuser was drinking before the act of violence occurred [5]. When examining inmates who were convicted of killing their intimate partner, 45% stated that they were drinking at the time of the homicide [5]. Additionally, this group had an average blood alcohol concentration (BAC) of three times the legal limit. Knowing about this association can provide a tactful means to segue into the issue of safety and IPV if the patient reports that they or their partner indulges with alcohol in excess. Making this connection can be useful to identify IPV whenever making inquiries about alcohol and substance use.

It is likely worthwhile to investigate IPV among those seeking treatment for addiction. A patient who is being victimized may turn to drugs or alcohol to cope with abuse, and so IPV may be a foreseeable and preventable contributor to relapse.

Knowing the myriad health issues that are associated with IPV, healthcare providers are strategically and conveniently positioned to identify and help prevent future incidents. In the United States, IPV affects more than one in three women in the course of their lives [6]. As many as 20% of all adult women accessing primary care services screen positive for recent IPV [6]. However, IPV is often not explored during visits to the doctor's office (particularly primary care). Institute of Medicine (IOM) has identified IPV screening as a critical and necessary procedure for women of child-bearing age [6].

Several factors may contribute to this phenomenon. A provider may not be familiar with IPV or its vast medical consequences. Moreover, most care providers are under time constraints to complete a physical and history. Exploring a delicate topic such as IPV can be time-consuming and perhaps take multiple visits. To some providers, exploring IPV may be anathema to their business model of efficiency and profit (this can be especially true if IPV occurrence does not seem obvious). There are many complex ways intimate partner violence influences health. The direct effects are quite obvious. These effects include injury, disability, and loss of life. Indeed, death is a possible consequence of intimate partner violence. From 1976 to 1996, 30% of all murdered women were killed by an intimate partner [7]. It is important to recognize that homicide is a leading cause of pregnancy-associated deaths [7].

Many symptoms that were given by victims of domestic violence were similar to the symptoms of anxiety and depression. Many of these are long-term [8]. This emphasizes the importance of screening. Intervention and prevention play an important role in stymying the negative impact of intimate partner violence [8].

Naturally, a provider may treat the patient symptomatically and move on. However, even if a provider does suspect intimate partner violence, they may still neglect to explore it due to a sad reality: an unresponsive healthcare provider can perpetuate the cycle of silence further isolating women who suffered abuse, rape, and other assaults [9]. Unfortunately, the majority of women who have been abused, assaulted, or raped have not disclosed their experience with their doctor [9]. For example, only about 29% of women who experienced intimate partner violence have had a discussion with their doctor. Of the women who talked about intimate partner violence with their doctor, 74% of women initiated the conversation [9]. This is truly a sad commentary on the state of intimate partner violence screening. Due to embarrassment, shame, or discomfort, many doctors may not initiate this conversation. Women suffering from intimate partner violence are more likely to report that they have switched doctors (in the past 5 years). Usually, the reason given is "being dissatisfied with care" [9].

In an article in *Social Science and Medicine* (1997) entitled "Domestic violence and mental health: correlates and conundrums within and across cultures," the concept of marital rape is explored. A case involving a married woman in Mexico is illustrated. The woman was forced to have sex with her husband. He used violence to obtain forceful sex from her. In addition, her husband has expressed views that "as his wife, she belongs to him and so he has the right to enjoy her whenever he desires." This began after a miscarriage. Her husband was of the opinion that she was faulty and could not bear children. He lashed out due to his underlying entitlement to both sex and offspring [10]. Long after her bruises had healed, the women mentioned had to summon the courage to complain to her doctor of a heaviness or "pain" in her heart [10].

As the community/society becomes increasingly more diverse, those in healthcare should be sensitive to culture attitudes toward domestic violence. Often, an abuser will use cultural norms to justify their continued perpetration of violence and coercive control. Acts that often fall under this umbrella of "cultural norms" are marital rape, dowry-related deaths, and exposure to STIs [10].

A study by Gremillion and Kanof entitled "Overcoming barriers to physician involvement in identifying and referring victims of domestic violence" from the *Annals of Emergency Medicine* found that 31% of patients who reported functional gastrointestinal disorders had a history of rape or incest [11].

Healthcare providers should not make the assumption that if no injury is evident, the patient is not a victim. Some presentations that may raise a healthcare professional's index of suspicion include [12]:

- Hypervigilance.
- Multiple doctor visits, either with or without injuries.
- Low self-esteem/low self-worth.
- Presenting with delay after an injury was sustained.
- Injuries to multiple areas on the body.
- Injuries in different stages of healing.
- History of substance use/self-medication.
- An injury is noted on a pregnant woman (physical abuse of a pregnant woman usually involves the abdomen or breasts).
- Mental health complaints: anxiety, depression, PTSD, or suicidal ideation.
- Headache.
- Gastrointestinal complaints.

Hopefully, increased awareness and efforts by clinicians such as this book will highlight the need for more screening.

The opportunity for intervention is great, but so, too, is the chance that intimate partner violence will go undiscovered and uncorrected. Not every victim of abuse openly discloses this information. There are many barriers keeping a victim from disclosing intimate partner violence. It is common that many victims often fail to recognize their partner's behavior as abusive. Even more regrettably, many victims of abuse feel as though they are the reason for their partner's abusive behavior. It is this self-blame, coupled with social isolation, that can skew a victim's perspective on what is abuse. Their partner's abusive behavior often is normalized as appropriate and may keep the victim from seeking help or sharing experiences with others. As will be reiterated throughout this book, it is important to note that abuse can be verbal or economic or involve emotional manipulation and coercion (as well as physical or sexual assault). Furthermore, most victims of abuse report an overwhelming sense of shame associated with them being in such a situation.

It may represent a great perceived failure and inadequacy on their part and make them reluctant to share. If the victim has been in this current abusive relationship for a prolonged period, there may be a fear that the length of the relationship delegitimizes the severity of abuse. If the relationship has continued for many years, then it may create the perception that "things are not that bad."

Another barrier that may keep a victim of intimate partner violence from disclosing abuse is the context and setting of the visit. If the victim is seeing a new and unfamiliar provider, they may be less likely to disclose abuse. If the patient feels as though there will be no follow up with the same provider, they may feel that their complaints will be wasted on someone they are likely to never see again.

Regarding the context and setting of the visit, the care provider should consider who may be accompanying the victim. The victim may be accompanied by a friend or family member and feel shame disclosing abuse while with them. Even more troubling, the victim may be accompanied by the perpetrator of abuse. If the abusive partner is the one who brings them to treatments or office visits, the victim may fear not being brought to follow-ups. Naturally, the risk of losing a tie to a particular provider or treatment for a chronic ailment could serve as a deterrent to disclose abuse.

Often overt threats from the perpetrator of abuse have been made to the victim. These threats can be of further or more severe harm to the victim. The perpetrator of abuse may have threatened to do harm to their children or themselves if disclosure of abuse was ever made.

Yet another consideration that may contribute to a victim's fear of disclosure is the fear of the consequences brought on by disclosure. They may not want their abuser to be harmed. This may happen through retaliatory methods taken on by the victim's family and friends. They may fear police involvement. This may stem from the fear that their partner may be arrested or jailed or that their private affairs may become public. The victim may be financially dependent on the abuser and may risk the loss of their home. They may be uncertain about the fate of their children or the abusive partner. This uncertainty may keep them from disclosing abuse. This can be especially troublesome in the formal setting of a hospital or doctor's office where notes are taken and records are kept. In order to set up a reassuring environment, it is important to discuss confidentiality and also the limits of confidentiality. It is important for a healthcare provider to be mindful of all these possible deterrents that victims may face before disclosing abuse and to address them as appropriate.

Being mindful of the emotional turmoil that can be associated with disclosing abuse, it is important to create a comfortable supportive environment for the victim. Remember abuse is a difficult thing to share. It is important that the care provider take adequate measures to ensure privacy. A victim may be put off if ancillary medical staff are nearby. As mentioned before, persons accompanying the victim may cause them discomfort in sharing such sensitive issues. The healthcare provider should attempt to speak to the victim privately. It is important to assess how quiet the interview area is. It may be necessary that the provider and victim go to a separate area so as not to be overheard or disrupted. Healthcare providers should take an active approach in addressing the issue of abuse. It is necessary to ask specific questions about abuse rather than vague inquiries.

The healthcare provider should assure the victim of abuse that they are here to listen to the victim talk. It is important never to push someone into revealing domestic abuse. Rather it is better to create assurances that the discussion can be had if and when the victim is ready. Not every individual will be open to discussing the topic. It may be prudent to consider taking gradual steps toward building rapport and facilitating conversation. It is important to make the person feel comfortable returning and continuing at a later date if need be. The care provider should ask if the victim of abuse would prefer to speak to someone else. For example, female abuse victims may feel better speaking to female care providers. If there is the need for an interpreter, use an official interpreter. The use of the victim's family or friends may keep the victim from being forthright due to the fears regarding stigma and privacy detailed earlier. Intimate partner violence among immigrant populations will be disused at length in other chapters. However, it is important to note, whenever encountering people from diverse cultures and backgrounds, abuse should never be viewed as normal or appropriate.

When asking about abuse, a care provider should frame their questions in a context that avoids stigma and judgment. Questions can be posed in routine social screening regarding various issues that may impact the health of the person in question. It is okay for a healthcare provider to express concern; however, they should never become accusatory or force disclosure of abuse. A healthcare provider should accept a denial of experiencing abuse as valid and continue to offer support. If abuse is revealed, then appropriate steps can be taken. Let the victim know that they are believed and that their suffering and concern are valid. The healthcare provider should inform the victim that abuse is common and that they are not alone in their suffering.

Most importantly, the point should be made that they deserve a safe life free of domestic violence and that this outcome can be achieved.

A provider should inquire if there are children in the household. If so, what is the status of their safety? There are health consequences for children who witness and/or experience abuse. Be sure to offer supportive information such as hotline numbers and support agencies. Often victims are exceedingly fearful of their partner and may not be able to take many printed documents with them. If possible, a healthcare provider should offer a small concise card with valuable information and numbers on it so that this item may be easily concealed if necessary. If a healthcare provider suspects intimate partner abuse, they should pass on the information to the person (during the patient encounter) regardless if there is disclosure of abuse. The victim may make use of it at a later date. A healthcare provider should not demand that the victim leave the abusive partner. The victim may not be safe if they leave the abuser. They may fear to live alone or could be financially tied to the perpetrator of abuse. They may still love the abuser.

Indeed, transitioning out of an abusive relationship can be a long process. Many life-changing concessions must be made. The victim likely will need time to plan before executing change. The healthcare provider should provide continuous support along the way. Until the abuse is resolved, strategies should be made to ensure the victim's safety and the safety of their children (if there are any). A safety plan can be made. This plan may serve to guide the victim while experiencing abuse in a relationship.

A safety plan is a well thought out course of action designed to help increase safety and decrease harm in an abusive environment/relationship. The healthcare provider and victim should discuss important phone numbers to keep in mind. If the victim were to leave home, where are a few places they could stay? What items would be needed if the victim leaves? Are these items already packed? Can the victim save money and store money? As mentioned before the perpetrators of abuse are often controlling. Documents, money, and extra clothes may need to be stored with someone else. Is there a person to fill that role in the victim's life? Has the victim shared these plans with their children?

When a victim shares abuse or injury with the healthcare provider, this data should be thoroughly documented. This information may be used later in legal proceedings regarding divorce, child custody, or restraining orders.

In closing, healthcare providers are often the first people to interact with a victim of abuse. This may be the rare chance a victim of intimate partner violence may have to receive help from a professional. Survivors of domestic abuse often need someone to ask about their relationship as a way to facilitate disclosure of abuse.

A victim of intimate partner violence is often under a tremendous stress burden. This stress burden can lead to very real physical manifestations that are often inscrutable and treatment resistant (if the root cause is never identified). Furthermore, some physical ailments are the direct cause of physical trauma. Yes, a bone can be set and a wound can be stitched. However, if a guided path to safety is not provided, abuse will likely continue. It befalls the healthcare provider to remain vigilant. It is often the goal of providers to be expert in their examination skills and history gathering. However, we must be mindful that a guarded secret may be the cause of untold suffering.

No longer should the simple designation of girlfriend, boyfriend, husband, or wife be unconditionally synonymous with a guardian who is forever absolved from causing a patient harm. If disclosure of abuse is given, a healthcare provider should foster validation and trust while being nonjudgmental. The healthcare provider's role is to provide the victimized patient with support and access to both information and safety. As with most social issues, IPV exists in a complex and emotional realm. It is not the role of the provider to force the patients' hand. Instead give them the tools, insight, and support needed to thoroughly and honestly examine their individual circumstance. Hopefully, the healthcare provider can deliver them to the realization that no one deserves to be victimized. Through their own autonomy and decision-making, they will remove themselves from the situation and with it gain dignity, confidence, self-reliance, and safety. Lastly, while maintaining a safe and sensitive environment, a healthcare professional should not forget to address their medical issues as well.

References

1. Sarkar NN. The impact of intimate partner violence on women's reproductive health and pregnancy outcome. J Obstet Gynaecol. 2008;28(3):266–71.

2. Feder GS, Hutson M, Ramsay J, Taket AR. Women exposed to intimate partner violence: expectations and experiences when they encounter health care professionals: a meta-analysis of qualitative studies. Arch Intl Med. 2006;166(1):22–37.
3. Wuest J, Ford-Gilboe M, Merritt-Gray M, Varcoe C, Lent B, Wilk P, Campbell J. Abuse-related injury and symptoms of posttraumatic stress disorder as mechanisms of chronic pain in survivors of intimate partner violence. Pain Med. 2009;10(4):739–47.
4. Devries KM, Mak JY, Bacchus LJ, Child JC, Falder G, Petzold M, et al. Intimate partner violence and incident depressive symptoms and suicide attempts: a systematic review of longitudinal studies. PLoS Med. 2013;10(5):e1001439.
5. Fals-Stewart W, Kennedy C. Addressing intimate partner violence in substance-abuse treatment. J Subst Abus Treat. 2005;29(1):5–17.
6. McCall-Hosenfeld JS, Weisman CS, Perry AN, Hillemeier MM, Chuang CH. "I just keep my antennae out" how rural primary care physicians respond to intimate partner violence. J Interpers Violence. 2014;29(14):2670–94.
7. Plichta SB. Intimate partner violence and physical health consequences: policy and practice implications. J Interpers Violence. 2004;19(11):1296–323.
8. Coker AL, Smith PH, Bethea L, King MR, McKeown RE. Physical health consequences of physical and psychological intimate partner violence. Arch Fam Med. 2000;9(5):451–7.
9. Plichta SB, Falik M. Prevalence of violence and its implications for women's health. Womens Health Issues. 2001;11(3):244–58.
10. Fischbach RL, Herbert B. Domestic violence and mental health: correlates and conundrums within and across cultures. Soc Sci Med. 1997;45(8):1161–76.
11. Gremillion DH, Kanof EP. Overcoming barriers to physician involvement in identifying and referring victims of domestic violence. Ann Emerg Med. 1996;27(6):769–73.
12. Buel SM. Family violence: practical recommendations for physicians and the medical community. Womens Health Issues. 1995;5(4):158–72.

Intimate Partner Violence: The Law

3

Rahn Kennedy Bailey

In April 2018, the Office on Violence Against Women (OVW), an office within the US Department of Justice, changed the definition of domestic violence [1]. The administration's new definition has a narrower scope. The US Department of Justice's OVW has defined domestic violence as "felony or misdemeanor crimes of violence committed by a current or former spouse or intimate partner of the victim, by a person with whom the victim shares a child in common, by a person who is cohabitating with or has cohabitated with the victim as a spouse or intimate partner, by a person similarly situated to a spouse of the victim under the domestic or family violence laws of the jurisdiction receiving grant monies, or by any other person against an adult or youth victim who is protected from that person's acts under the domestic or family violence laws of the jurisdiction" [2]. This definition neglects other well-established aspects of domestic violence. Under this definition, domestic violence is limited to physical violence. Furthermore, it qualifies the level of physical violence as that which rises to the level of a felony or misdemeanor.

This new definition is troubling. Coercive control, threats, verbal, and psychological abuse are totally absent from this definition. This book has pointed out how such abusive tactics can negatively impact a victim's quality of life. It is often the coercive control and threats that create an atmosphere of helplessness. We should not neglect the unseen abuse. A victim's self-confidence and personal worth is often ruined by nonphysical abuse [3]. It is paramount that the other major components of domestic violence are not forgotten in the legal or social realm. Often, these nonphysical actions can be more difficult for victims to deal with [3].

In years past, intimate partner violence (IPV) was viewed as a private matter. Society and the justice system alike tended to hold the overarching belief that such issues (private) did not warrant official attention or intervention. Thankfully, this

R. K. Bailey (✉)
Department of Psychiatry, Charles R. Drew University of Medicine and Science, Los Angeles, CA, USA
e-mail: rahnkbaileymd@comcast.net

R. K. Bailey (ed.), *Intimate Partner Violence*,
https://doi.org/10.1007/978-3-030-55864-2_3

view has largely changed, and the widespread ill effects of IPV are appreciated and given full credence as real legal and public health concerns. In this chapter, we will explore how the law (in the United States) has progressed to reflect this change in the social collective.

Through advocacy and publicity, attention and awareness have been brought to the issue of IPV. This increased attention and awareness has in turn led to changes within the justice system. Victims of IPV now have the access to protective court orders and other legal protections [4]. These protections reflect a change in the justice system that has occurred over the past 40 years [5]. However, not all of the changes in the justice system have led to progress. Currently, there are two schools of thought regarding IPV. Some believe it is the duty of the justice system to address the issue of IPV for it is a social ill. Others have taken to passive and quiet resignation. The second school of thought believes that victims of IPV are uncooperative in the role to help combat domestic violence.

Some in the criminal justice system have indeed grown frustrated by the apparent apathy sometimes shown by victims of IPV. Advocates for victims of domestic violence point to theoretical models such as "the power and control wheel" to explain some victims' hesitancy to seek intervention. The power and control wheel is a description of how the use of abuse and threat of violence can control a victim's life [6]. Those in the justice system are now becoming more aware of the circumstances that may make a victim act unexpectedly amidst the prospect of escaping an abusive relationship. Thus, the law has adapted itself to allow intervention with minimal participation by victims [5, 6]. These changes in policy now yield more allowance for prosecutors, judges, policymakers, and police to protect victims regardless of whether they (the victims) express wishes to the contrary [5, 6]. This dynamic often makes litigating domestic violence cases complex and difficult.

In the United States what has been the history of the law and domestic violence? During the early Colonial period, British law was the standard. The law allowed for husbands to control their wives through means of "domestic chastisement" [7]. That is to say, a man was permitted to use corporal punishment against his wife. Until the mid-1900s, the so-called rule of thumb prevailed. Under this dictum, a man is permitted to physically discipline his wife so long as he did not use an implement "thicker than his thumb" [8]. In the case of Joyner v. Joyner, 59 N.C. 322 (1862), the ruling read "holding that the law gives the husband power to use such a degree of force as is necessary to make the wife behave herself" [9]. Such sentiments no doubt would seem egregious today. Matters of domestic violence continued to be held as a private matter that does not need any intervention by legal authorities. In the 1960s, people became more socially conscious. Efforts were made to provide shelters for abused women. However, even during this time, women had little legal recourse. Not until the 1970s and 1980s did statutes proliferate establishing victims' rights to pursue civil injunctions against batterers to protect them from further violence and establish ground rules for separation.

In 2014, the Bureau of Labor Statistics estimated that over 600,000 acts of violent crime were perpetrated by an intimate partner. In 2014 the rate of IPV was 2.4 per 1000 [10]. Severe physical violence such as being struck with blunt objects, being kicked or hit, or being burned intentionally was experienced by an estimated 22.3% of women and 14.0% of men during their lifetimes [11].

Most of the domestic violence laws are state laws. The Violence Against Women Act was the first federal statute aimed at gender-related violence. In 1994, this act created funding for agencies that offer support for victims of abuse. It also appropriated funds for domestic violence research [12].

At the state level, there is no unified classification of domestic violence law. It may be in the criminal or civil domain. Usually, statutes place assault, battery, stalking, rape against a family member, or intimate partner in the realm of domestic violence offenses.

In this book intimate partner violence among immigrant communities is discussed. It has been addressed that a common deterrent for abused immigrants from contacting the authorities is the fear of deportation [13]. In the 2000 reiteration of the Violence Against Women Act, the Battered Immigrant Protection Act was introduced. This provision created U-visas and T-visas that provided protections to undocumented victims of abuse and human trafficking. By granting victims visas, the fear of deportation is eliminated, and cooperation with authorities is drastically unhindered. U-visas grant a victim the ability to work and live in the United States. Additionally, any pending litigation regarding immigration or deportation could potentially be dismissed [14]. The requirements for U-visas are that a visa petitioner has been a victim of abuse as a result of a crime (in the United States) and the victim has knowledge of the crime and will help in the investigation/prosecution of said crime. Similar conditions are in place for granting T-visas to victims of human trafficking. However, the requirement to assist in the investigation of trafficking crimes may be lifted if the participation is considered too traumatizing for the victim. If a victim obtains a U-visa, the holder's immediate family may then also gain the benefits and protections of the visa. Though these visas were created to quell fears of deportation and allow for accurate reporting of abuse, many immigrants are still unaware of these safeguards. Unfortunately, some perpetrators of abuse may exploit this ignorance of the law to prevent their victim from reporting or separating.

In the 2013 rendition of the Violence Against Women Act, more inclusive language was added to provide protection to the LGBTQ community. There are unique challenges faced by people in the LBGTQ community regarding aid [15]. For example, battered women's shelters may not be accommodating to adult men or trans women who are the victim of IPV. The Violence Against Women Act ensures access to all services for victims of domestic violence. Additionally, it has provided funding to aid the LGBTQ community.

In 2000, the Violence Against Women Act was broadened to include expansive protections for Native American People. There are some alarming statistics regarding IPV and the Native American population. 39–79% of Native American women will experience IPV during their lifetime [14, 16, 17]. Violence against Native American women tends to be perpetrated by non-native men.

This odd statistic is due to the marriages of Native American and non-native people. In 2013, the Violence Against Women Act allowed for tribes to enforce laws regarding domestic violence regarding a non-native. Previous to this, tribal courts would not prosecute a non-native (even if the non-native committed a crime against a native on tribal grounds). There have been concessions allowing tribes the ability to honor criminal sanctions brought forth by any other state or native territory [18].

There has been some criticism of the Violence Against Women Act. First, some people believe that the 2013 version of the Violence Against Women Act has caused more underreporting of abuse. Underreporting may have started to take place with the institution of automatic arrest policies. It is thought that many people may not want their abuser to be arrested and may not report abuse. Second, although many people applaud what the legislation has done to help victims of abuse, critics are quick to point out that not much regarding the prevention of abuse is addressed [19].

Another area of concern regarding victims of IPV is the number of homicides. Statistically, 2/3 of women who were killed by a firearm were killed by an intimate partner. In the United States, the Gun Control Act is federal legislation that controls firearm owners and manufactures. In 1996 this law was modified with the Lautenberg Amendment. This amendment introduced further restrictions regarding the ownership and possession of firearms. The act extended gun prohibitions to non-felons if one of two criteria is met. If an individual has been convicted of a misdemeanor crime of domestic violence or if they have pending restraining order, then they are prohibited from gun ownership [20].

Battered woman syndrome is a theory that seeks to describe the mental state of victims of abuse. The condition describes a mental state brought upon by stress and repeated trauma, in which a victim becomes apathetic and depressed and remains with the abuser despite the negative consequences of the relationship [21]. There are thought to be three major tenants in battered woman syndrome. First, the victim of abuse believes the abuse is their own fault. Second, there is a sense of fear for safety and fear of future acts of violence. Lastly, there is the belief that retaliatory violence (by the abuser) is inevitable if disclosure of abuse is made. Sufferers of battered woman syndrome are often so fearful of their abuser that taking action is often too daunting [22]. This becomes even more problematic in a courtroom setting. Often due to overwhelming and irrational fear, battered women will not testify against the perpetrator of abuse. Battered woman syndrome has been used in litigation as an explanation for why a victim of abuse may kill or seriously injure their abusive partner. Battered woman syndrome provides a perspective into the victim's mind frame and may provide justification for their action. The argument often presented in court is that a victim is in fear of imminent and inescapable danger. Thus, the action that may have injured or killed their abuser is justified, and the victim should not be culpable [23].

Battered woman syndrome has been used and accepted in the legal community. However, it is not without criticism. A major argument against the battered woman testimony is that it paints a picture of a person who is overcome and does not possess the ability to reason.

This can be problematic because the victim can be seen as disordered and may lose custody of her children [24]. If the victim has shown any behavior that is anathema to the jury's idea of what a helpless, overcome, and irrational battered woman should be, this could ruin her case. The main obstacle of this defense tactic is that few women perfectly personify the ideal image of a battered woman syndrome put forth by the court.

Another criticism of battered woman syndrome (for consistency with the other mentions) and its' use in court is that it is not inclusive. Many LGBTQ people and males suffer emotional consequences of abuse, yet their situation may not be viewed with the same mitigation or sympathy [25].

On the state level, progress has been made regarding male and LGBTQ persons and the law. Forty-two states have laws regarding domestic abuse that is either gender-neutral or are LGBTQ inclusive. Though most states still retain the term "battered women" and its narrow definition, some progressive states have adopted the term "battered spouses." However, the battered spouse syndrome defense has not seen much success in court. Many in society are still skeptical of power imbalances (deficits) males and LGBTQ people may have in a relationship.

Therefore, many prejudices and misconceptions still hinder the use of the battered women syndrome defense. During a trial in 1988, the battered woman defense was used regarding the case of Annette Green. After years of abuse, Green killed her same-sex partner. In this case, all jurors believed the relationship was abusive; however, they did not accept battered woman syndrome as a defense and convicted her. Cases like this highlight how the public, and importantly, a jury, views abuse and self-defense in homosexual vs. heterosexual relationships [26].

There are many laws in place that require healthcare professionals to report injuries that have resulted from a crime. However, only a few states require health professionals to report injuries that they suspect have resulted from domestic violence. California is a state that requires mandatory reporting of suspected domestic violence. Those in favor of the law have argued that this type of enforced reporting brings more people to justice and helps curtail abuse.

However, opponents of the law argue that mandatory reporting of domestic violence naturally leads to abusers preventing victims from getting health care. The American Medical Association opposes mandatory reporting. California law directs healthcare providers to report suspected domestic violence abuse even if it is in opposition to the victim's desire or wishes. Furthermore, a physician can face fines of up to $1000 and/or up to 6 months imprisonment if they do not comply with reporting abuse [27].

What do victims of IPV think of mandatory reporting? A patient survey was part of an emergency department IPV intervention study and involved 12 emergency departments, randomly drawn from all midsized hospitals (20,000–40,000 patient visits annually) within 100 miles of San Francisco, CA, and Pittsburgh, PA [24]. The study yielded mixed results. The study showed that 44.3% of recently abused female emergency department patients were against mandatory reporting of domestic violence to police. The study pointed to some of the reasons why a victim may be against mandatory reporting. The victim may fear the abuser or fear the separation of their family. However, 55.7% of participants in the study supported mandatory reporting [27]. This may allow the victim to avoid retaliation from their abuser. Indeed, they may get police attention and bring about investigation without having to personally betray, blame, accuse, and upset their intimate partner.

Records

In the National Intimate Partner and Sexual Violence Survey, United States, 2011, the lifetime and 12-month prevalence of rape by an intimate partner for women were examined. The survey estimated a lifetime prevalence of rape to be 8.8%. The 12-month prevalence was 0.8%. The survey found that 0.8% of men reported rape by an intimate partner in their lifetime. 12-month prevalence of rape for men could not be ascertained in a statistically reliable way due to low reports [11].

The National Intimate Partner and Sexual Violence Survey, United States, 2011, provided information on severe physical violence as well. Severe violence in the form of acts such as the following were suffered by an estimated 22.3% of women and 14.0% of men (during their lifetimes):

- Struck by a weapon
- Being kicked or punched
- Intentionally burned

An estimated 2.3% of women and 2.1% of men endured such acts of violence, at the hands of an intimate partner, in the 12 months before taking the survey [11].

Per the National Crime Victimization Survey (NCVS) 2014, the rate of intimate partner violence has not decreased significantly. Looking at a 1-year period (2013–2014), the rate of IPV committed by current of former partners (spouses or girl/boyfriend) remained at 4.2 per 1000 [10].

In fact, violence is the leading cause of injury for women aged 15–44 [28].

Additional Benefits Brought Forth by the Violence Against Women Act

The Violence Against Women Act allowed the appropriation of 1.6 billion USD to improve response to intimate partner violence. This was done through strengthening the enforcement of existing laws and the implementation of new federal laws. Funding was allocated to social programs, education, and prevention. Another important result of the Violence Against Women Act was the establishment of a new office within the US Department of Justice. This new office's primary purpose was/is to address the issue of violence against women. Thus, the government took a national approach to solving a national problem [29, 30].

With updates to the Violence Against Women Act, laws were extended to protect more relationships. Consideration was taken for relationships that function as a typical marriage would. That is to say, couples are interdependent, share finances, and are in an intimate relationship. This notion is known as "marriage mimicry." In some areas, the judicial system has taken a broad approach to the issue. By adopting this kind of model when interpreting the law, more people can fall under protections [25].

Society still has to evolve in its thinking when regarding domestic violence. Often, law enforcement can be uncertain how to proceed with cases involving same-sex individuals. The perpetrator is often thought to be the larger of the two individuals involved. If the case involves a heterosexual couple, it is often assumed the male is the aggressor [15]. Again, this is likely due to law enforcement making generalizations. Furthermore, transgender individuals may be gender misidentified and incorrectly assumed to be a perpetrator or victim accordingly. Further still, law enforcement may think that simply by being transgender, the individual is a reprobate and thus culpable [15].

Civil Law and Intimate Partner Violence

All 50 states have procedures for victims of domestic violence to obtain civil protection orders. A civil protection order is a court order that offers protection to a victim of IPV. Each state has its own criteria that qualify an individual for a civil protection order. Violation of a civil protection order is a criminal offense in all 50 states.

Domestic violence and its influence in child custody will be discussed throughout this book. Children and their welfare are major influences in a victim's decision-making process. Lack of financial support or the risk of separation from their children may keep a victim with their abuser. Many jurisdictions consider the issue of domestic violence when considering child custody cases. Most states impose varying degrees of child custody limitations on perpetrators of abuse. Some states, like Nebraska, New York, and California, have denied child custody to the victim. Those in favor of this view claim that the victim failed to protect the child from witnessing abuse and so was negligent in their parental duties.

In closing, this chapter has highlighted some of the legislation that has been instituted in the United States regarding the issue of domestic violence. Bias and cultural attitudes still exist and can have an influence on juries and judges alike. The interplay of emotion, family, and finance is complex, and there are myriad reasons why a victim would stay with their abuser. Without sensitivity to this dynamic, the way legal proceedings are adjudicated may be unfair to victims of abuse.

Individuals who are in the LGBTQ community may not enjoy the fullest legal protections when compared to those in heterosexual relationships. However, the trend is moving toward a deeper understating of IPV and its far-reaching effects on very diverse groups of people. Thus there is optimism that the current laws shall evolve to be all inclusive.

References

1. https://www.independent.co.uk/news/world/americas/trump-domestic-abuse-sexual-assault-definition-womens-rights-justice-department-a8744546.html?fbclid=IwAR0qLzMKZA9FB9jr7y3MtY05iGHem9GDdia98ZDRw3E6sSSxLsLPj69FoJ4. Last accessed 22 Sept 2019.
2. https://www.justice.gov/ovw/domestic-violence. Last accessed 22 Sept 2019.
3. Williamson E. Living in the world of the domestic violence perpetrator: negotiating the unreality of coercive control. Violence Against Women. 2010;16(12):1412–23.
4. Schneider EM. Domestic violence law reform in the twenty-first century: looking back and looking forward. Family Law Q. 2008;42(3):353–63.

5. Kohn L. The justice system and domestic violence: engaging the case but divorcing the victim. N York U Rev Law Soc Change. 2008;32(2):2012–134.
6. Rankine J, Percival T, Finau E, Hope LT, Kingi P, Peteru MC, et al. Pacific peoples, violence, and the power and control wheel. J Interpers Violence. 2017;32(18):2777–803.
7. Murray VH. A comparative survey of the historic civil, common, and American Indian tribal law responses to domestic violence. Okla City UL Rev. 1998;23:433.
8. Kelly HA. Rule of thumb and the Folklaw of the Husband's stick. J Legal Educ. 1994;44:341.
9. Pavlidakis A. Mandatory arrest: past its prime. Santa Clara L Rev. 2009;49:1201.
10. Truman JL, Langton L. Criminal victimization, U.S. Department of Justice Bureau of Justice Statistics 2. 2014. http://www.bjs.gov/content/pub/pdf/cv14.pdf.
11. Breiding MJ. Prevalence and characteristics of sexual violence, stalking, and intimate partner violence victimization—National Intimate Partner and Sexual Violence Survey, United States, 2011. MMWR Surveill Summ. 2014;63(8):1–18.
12. Orloff LE, Kaguyutan JV. Offering a helping hand: legal protections for battered immigrant women: a history of legislative responses. Am. UJ Gender Soc Poly L. 2002;10:95.
13. Raj A, Silverman J. Violence against immigrant women: the roles of culture, context, and legal immigrant status on intimate partner violence. Violence Against Women. 2002;8(3):367–98.
14. Bardavid D, Chiarolanzio M, Strittmater A. Domestic violence. Georgetown J Gender Law. 2016;17(1):211–46.
15. Morrison AM. Queering domestic violence to straighten out criminal law: what might happen when queer theory and practice meet criminal law's conventional responses to domestic violence. S Cal Rev L Women's Stud. 2003;13:81.
16. Malcoe LH, Duran BM, Montgomery JM. Socioeconomic disparities in intimate partner violence against Native American women: a cross-sectional study. BMC. 2004;2(1):20.
17. Fairchild DG, Fairchild MW, Stoner S. Prevalence of adult domestic violence among women seeking routine care in a Native American health care facility. Am J Public Health. 1998;88(10):1515–7.
18. Bent-Goodley TB. Culture and domestic violence: transforming knowledge development. J Interpers Violence. 2005;20(2):195–203.
19. Modi MN, Palmer S, Armstrong A. The role of Violence Against Women Act in addressing intimate partner violence: a public health issue. J Women's Health. 2014;23(3):253–9.
20. Nathan AJ. At the intersection of domestic violence and guns: the public interest exception and the Lautenberg amendment. Cornell L Rev. 1999;85:822.
21. Appleton W. The battered woman syndrome. Ann Emerg Med. 1980;9(2):84–91.
22. Astin MC, Lawrence KJ, Foy DW. Posttraumatic stress disorder among battered women: risk and resiliency factors. Violence Vict. 1993;8(1):17.
23. Ono E. Reformulating the use of battered woman syndrome testimonies in Canadian law: implications for social work practice. Affilia. 2017;32(1):24–36.
24. Cahn NR. Civil images of battered women: the impact of domestic violence on child custody decisions. Vand L Rev. 1991;44:1041.
25. Colker R. Marriage mimicry: the law of domestic violence. Wm Mary L Rev. 2005;47:1841.
26. Little S. Challenging changing legal definitions of family in same-sex domestic violence. Hastings Women's LJ. 2008;19:259.
27. Rodriguez MA, McLoughlin E, Nah G, Campbell JC. Mandatory reporting of domestic violence injuries to the police: what do emergency department patients think? JAMA. 2001;286(5):580–3.
28. Shargel JR. In defense of the civil rights remedy of the violence against women act. Yale LJ. 1996;106:1849.
29. Runge RR. The evolution of a national response to violence against women. Hastings Women's LJ. 2013;24:429.
30. Weissman DM. Gender-based violence as judicial anomaly: between the truly national and the truly local. BCL Rev. 2000;42:1081. http://lawdigitalcommons.bc.edu/bclr/vol42/iss5/2.

Intimate Partner Violence: Law Enforcement

4

Mallory Williams and Rahn Kennedy Bailey

Intimate partner violence involves controlling behavior perpetrated by an individual that causes physical or emotional damage and incites fear. The abuser commonly controls or changes the behavior of an intimate partner through physical violence, coercion, threats, and isolation [1]. Many victims often have difficulty in both obtaining help and severing a relationship. When a perpetrator of abuse is an officer of the law (particularly a well-connected one), seeking help from authorities can become especially daunting.

Does Intimate Partner Violence Occur Among Individuals in Law Enforcement?

Studies that examined the prevalence of intimate partner violence (IPV) in the adult married and cohabitating populations in the United States found rates that ranged from 8% to 20% [1]. Working in law enforcement can be tremendously stressful. Some individuals may be present at gruesome crime scenes [1]. While enforcing the law, officers may encounter violent resistance [1]. Some argue that the very training that many law enforcement agents undergo contributes to IPV perpetration. In the article, "Intimate Partner Violence Within Law Enforcement Families," Anderson and Lo emphasize a particular aspect of police training that could contribute to

M. Williams
Howard University Hospital, Washington, DC, USA

Howard University College of Medicine, Washington, DC, USA

Howard University National Center of Excellence for Trauma & Violence Prevention, Washington, DC, USA

R. K. Bailey (✉)
Department of Psychiatry, Charles R. Drew University of Medicine and Science, Los Angeles, CA, USA
e-mail: rahnkbaileymd@comcast.net

R. K. Bailey (ed.), *Intimate Partner Violence*,
https://doi.org/10.1007/978-3-030-55864-2_4

increased IPV rates. They point to how police are "trained to dominate." Physical and psychological domination is taught through the use of posturing and verbal intimation [1]. These learned skills can then be used to dominate both while on the job and in a domestic setting. The display of dominance is then positively reinforced throughout an officer's career. This may create difficulty in leaving this outlook. Carrying it home can lead to use of intimidation and control at home and/or in a relationship [1]. Furthermore, the adoption of an authoritarian personality is suggested to be linked to the possibility of perpetrating intimate partner abuse. The matter of authoritarianism and IPV has been explored in a few studies. These studies have found links between authoritarianism and domestic violence.

In the study, Intimate Partner Violence Within Law Enforcement Families, Anderson and Lo examined self-reported IPV perpetration among full-time law enforcement officers within the Baltimore City Police Department. They found that 9% reported intimate violence perpetration. These incidences of violence (becoming physically aggressive) corresponded to high work-related stress [1].

The problem seems to be more widespread among law enforcement. Two studies in the 1990s (Johnson, 1991b; Neidig, Russell, & Seng, 1992) found that 40% of police families had occurrences of IPV [2, 3].

The threat of injury or loss of life can add considerable work-related stress. Increased work-related stress is a suggested reason for increased prevalence of intimate partner violence seen among law enforcement [4].

Authoritarian personalities expect submission, reverence, and subordination to be given to authority figures [5]. In the context of an intimate relationship, this can be quite problematic. Often successful relationships require varying degrees of compromise, diplomacy, and empathy. However, when one partner requires blind obedience from the other partner, abusive tactics may be used to ensure that they continue to receive it [6].

Some factors have been identified as increasing the likelihood of IPV perpetration among officers. These are as follows:

- Working shifts that are at odd times
- Working long shifts
- Sleep deprivation
- Not taking time off
- Dissatisfaction with job
- Being on patrol
- Working as a narcotics officer
- Poor coping skills [6]

In the face of real workplace danger, the establishment of dominance may be appropriate (perhaps necessary to safety). Unfortunately, it is often a maladaptive strategy when used on intimate partners [7, 8].

In 1991, efforts were made to link workplace stress with IPV. After surveying 728 police officers, Johnson reported before US Congress that 40% had "lost control" and used violence against their spouse [9]. These numbers exceed the much lower rates that have been touted by studies conducted entirely within law enforcement agencies [9]. However, attention and action have been taken regarding the issue of IPV among law enforcement officials. The Omnibus Consolidated Appropriations Act of 1996 (Lautenberg Amendment) addressed a component of domestic violence and law enforcement. This amendment made it illegal for (anyone, including but not limited to) officers of the law who were/are convicted of domestic violence crimes to possess a firearm [9]. The law's scope allowed it to be retroactive, thus prohibiting officers/anyone previously convicted of domestic violence from legally carrying a firearm. This had the large-scale effect of causing multiple law enforcement agencies to examine the domestic violence history of their officers.

Another reason given that may contribute to the creation of an environment that lends itself to IPV perpetration (by police) is the so-called cultural isolationism. Organizations often develop unique cultures and subcultures that dictate what is appropriate behavior in the context of that work environment [9]. Interestingly, police subculture tends to promote ideals lending toward control, authority, solidarity, and isolation [9]. These values are also a cornerstone of maintaining coercive control in an abusive domestic relationship. Police often have to treat the majority of encounters with civilians as potentially threatening. The use of caution and suspicion can create a perception of inherent rivalry and antagonism between police and individuals in the community [9]. This is often coupled with the fact that many officers participate in shift work. This can make it hard to maintain close relationships and/or friendships with those outside the police community [9]. Cumulatively, this can create social cultural isolation.

According to a report by Bailey (1995), prior to age 40, much of a police officer's life is spent enshrouded in police subculture [10]. Not only does this serve to socially isolate officers; it also serves to build comradery among officers. Indeed, loyalty and comradery are often promoted and practiced. This can be quite helpful while on patrol. However, some officers have agreed not to testify against or openly expose the wrongdoing of another officer. This can lead to the potential for cover-ups of wrongdoings [9, 10]. This can create a unique situation when an intimate partner of an officer calls the police for help. In fact, an intimate partner of an officer who is familiar with police culture and comradery may elect not to involve the cops, perhaps, taking the view that nothing substantial will be done to deter the abusive partner. Departments may minimize the actions of their officers [11]. This can make the victim of violence at the hands of an officer an isolated and "invisible" victim.

There is also another consideration a victim in this situation must make. Not only is there the possibility that fellow officers may not intervene; there is the real possibility that a (futile) report to the police will only serve to anger the perpetrator and escalate their level of abuse. Furthermore, an officer may know where most, if not all, of the battered shelters are. This, coupled with an officer's likely familiarity with the judicial system, can easily dissuade a victim from taking action. Thus, a victim may choose divorce as a means to end the relationship. Though divorce rates among police officers are high, it remains unclear if violence plays a factor in separation.

In attempting to identify potential contributors to IPV perpetration, some have pointed to work-related "burnout." Burnout is the inability to physically or psychologically cope with the stress associated with work/work environment [12]. The likelihood of burnout increases when individuals deal with troubled communities or individuals and feel as though their efforts at work are not helping [13]. Shift work is another potential component to police life that is both psychically and psychologically taxing [13]. Emotional control and restraint is emphasized while on the job. This, coupled with aggression, may cause officers to lash out while at home. Domestic violence risk is increased if an officer takes to alcohol use as a coping mechanism [13].

Police training teaches individuals to take control of situations. Officers are rewarded for exhibiting control, dominance, and authority. Thus, officers become proficient at exhibiting physical and verbal tactics to dominate. There is some question as to whether workplace attitudes spillover into domestic life. In a survey among 728 officers and 479 spouses, the most frequent complaint reported was "inability to leave the job at work" [14]. Relationships between job demands, emotional exhaustion, and work-family conflict have been reported [15–17].

Have initiatives been taken to assist victims whose partners are in law enforcement? Alerting law enforcement is often the first of many steps taken to remedy domestic violence. Domestic violence-related calls to law enforcement remain the largest category of calls received by police [18].

There was a case that infamously illustrated the predicament abused partners of officers often face. Crystal Brame was in an abusive marriage. Her husband exhibited many of the characteristics of coercive control often exhibited by abusive partners. Crystal Brame had to ask permission to leave the household. The length of time she spent outside of the house was closely monitored. Her receipts were closely checked and accounted for. In addition, her husband was verbally abusive. He often disparaged her appearance calling her "fat" and "ugly" [19, 20]. He also psychologically abused her. He threatened her repeatedly and placed loaded guns to her head. He choked her multiple times. Her husband was David Brame, the Chief of Police in Tacoma, Washington [19, 20]. Studies have shown violence within police families to range from 22% to 41%. This is in the neighborhood of 2–4 times that of the general population [20]. Similar to other police families, the two lived in an abusive relationship that cycled from violence to perfuse apology by Chief Brame. Crystal told her husband she may go to the authorities if the abuse continued. However, he was dismissive saying "who are you going to call, one of my buddies?" [20]. Crystal did, however, make a formal complaint. The report was not only stifled internally, but the Assistant Police Chief began harassing Crystal [20]. After his wife filed for divorce, the two became estranged. However, this did not completely deter Chief Brame. He confronted his ex-wife (along with their two young children) in a strip mall. The chief shot and killed Crystal, and then he turned his weapon on himself (committing suicide). As seen with the case of the Brames, separation does not always end the cycle of abuse. In fact, some reports estimate that separated couples had three times more "severe violence" [20] relative to couples living together.

There are some factors that may allow an abusive officer to escape prosecution and punishment. During their work as an officer, an abuser may encounter and investigate domestic violence cases. This allows the abuser to become very knowledgeable on what domestic violence "typically" looks like. A savvy officer may adjust his pattern of violence in ways less likely to leave bruises (or at least typical or obvious ones) [20]. Escaping an abusive relationship is problematic and dangerous for any victim. Escape can be more problematic and dangerous for victims whose abusers are officers. There are few if any areas that are beyond an officer's ability to access [20]. In the course of doing their duty, an officer may have visited all the local battered women's shelters. This would give the officer intimate knowledge of the location and the day-to-day goings-on of the shelter. Furthermore, those who work at the shelter may come to look at the officer as a benevolent figure. His routine appearance there may not be questioned. This could make it easy for an officer to track down an estranged partner.

On-the-job experience with domestic violence may prompt officers to take particularly crafty measures to preemptively create an innocent persona that is beyond reproach. For example, an abusive officer may secretly file a domestic violence report against their partner. This creates the perception and, more importantly, legal documentation that the victim was/is "abusive" [21]. Thus, if violence could not be contained and the authorities were involved, there would already be previous complaints against the victim. In a case like this, the judicial system/law enforcement would likely support the officer/abuser. Interestingly, David Brame had a reputation as an advocate against domestic violence within his department [20, 21]. Having knowledge of domestic violence places officers at an advantage of preemptively fabricating incidences to tarnish the victim's reputation and/or credibility. For example, an officer may make it appear as though his partner is stalking him appearing to be afraid [21]. Thus, over time, the victim can appear to be unstable or violent. Again, if an investigation were to occur, it would be quite easy to side with the officer.

The Brame case is one of many murder-suicides attributed to work-related stress and domestic conflict observed among law enforcement officers [22]. Most domestic violence-related murder-suicides are done with an official service issued firearm [23].

This highlights how difficult it can be for victims whose abusive partners are in law enforcement. Training in/access to firearms and computer databases make an abusive officer particularly threatening and capable of profound control. Furthermore, the fraternal bond among many officers may make it difficult to escape or get any meaningful recourse. Indeed, the training and comradery may add to a sense of impunity that some officers may feel (emboldening them further). This could be a contributing factor to IPV perpetration among officers of the law. These stress-inducing work conditions tend to increase domestic disharmony [8]. Though some departments implement services to help officers deal with work-related stress, most of these services remain underutilized [24].

In conclusion, studies show that individuals in law enforcement tend to perpetrate domestic violence at rates greater than the general population. Certain skills that serve an officer well while on the job can make that individual particularly adroit at perpetrating IPV. Indeed, the ability to be authoritative, controlling, and psychologically intimidating can serve to protect the officer and the community at large. However, such tactics can be extraordinarily effective when used on an intimate partner. Throughout this book, the difficulty abused partners have when trying to escape an abusive relationship has been highlighted. The plight of a victim who is abused by an officer of the law can be particularly bleak. Police officers tend to be a tight-knit cohort. Many may be reluctant to use civil force against a fellow officer. Additionally, the resources an officer has allow them to easily stalk an estranged partner if they wish. Partners of law enforcement are a unique group of victims that can be especially isolated. Thus, this chapter was crafted to bring awareness to the circumstances these particular individuals face.

References

1. Anderson AS, Lo CC. Intimate partner violence within law enforcement families. J Interpers Violence. 2011;26(6):1176–93.
2. Johnson LB. Police officers: gender comparisons. The encyclopedia of police science. 2nd ed. New York: Garland; 1995. p. 591–8.
3. Neidig PH, Russell HE, Seng AF. Interspousal aggression in law enforcement families: a preliminary investigation. Police Stud Int Rev Police Dev. 1992;15:30.
4. Waters JA, Ussery W. Police stress: history, contributing factors, symptoms, and interventions. Policing Int J Police Strategies Manag. 2007;30(2):20.
5. Can SH, Hendy HM. Police stressors, negative outcomes associated with them and coping mechanisms that may reduce these associations. Police J. 2014;87(3):167–77.
6. Griffin SP, Bernard TJ. Angry aggression among police officers. Police Q. 2003;6(1):3–21.
7. Bonifacio P. Criminal justice and public safety. The psychological effects of police work: a psychodynamic approach. New York: Springer. 1991.
8. Roberts NA, Levenson RW. The remains of the workday: impact of job stress and exhaustion on marital interaction in police couples. J Marriage Fam. 2001;63(4):1052–67.
9. Johnson LB, Todd M, Subramanian G. Violence in police families: work-family spillover. J Family Violence. 2005;20(1):3–12.
10. Bailey WG, editor. The encyclopedia of police science. New York: Taylor & Francis; 1995.
11. Armacost BE. Organizational culture and police misconduct. George Washington Law Rev. 2004;72(3):453–546.
12. Gershon RR, Barocas B, Canton AN, Li X, Vlahov D. Mental, physical, and behavioral outcomes associated with perceived work stress in police officers. Criminal Justice Behav. 2009;36(3):275–89.
13. Swatt ML, Gibson CL, Piquero NL. Exploring the utility of general strain theory in explaining problematic alcohol consumption by police officers. J Criminal Justice. 2007;35(6):596–611.
14. Johnson LB. On the front lines: police stress and family well-being. In: Hearing before the select committee on children, youth, and families house of representatives: 102 congress first session 1991, vol. 20, p. 32.
15. Hall GB, Dollard MF, Tuckey MR, Winefield AH, Thompson BM. Job demands, work-family conflict, and emotional exhaustion in police officers: a longitudinal test of competing theories. J Occupational Organizational Psychol. 2010;83(1):237–50.
16. Aaron JD. Stress and coping in police officers. Police Q. 2000;3(4):438–50.
17. Beehr TA, Johnson LB, Nieva R. Occupational stress: coping of police and their spouses. J Organizational Behav. 1995;16(1):3–25.
18. Russell BL, Pappas N. Officer involved domestic violence: a future of uniform response and transparency. Int J Police Sci Manag. 2018;20(2):134–42.

19. Stinson PM, Liederbach J. Fox in the henhouse: a study of police officers arrested for crimes associated with domestic and/or family violence. Criminal Justice Policy Rev. 2013;24(5):601–25.
20. Ammons J. Batterers with badges: officer-involved domestic violence. Women Law J. 2004;90:28.
21. Lonsway K, Wetendorf DE, Conis P. Lessons learned from Tacoma: the problem of police officer domestic violence. Law Enforcement Executive Forum. 2003;3(5):27–36.
22. Violanti JM. Homicide-suicide in police families: aggression full circle. Int J Emerg Mental Health. 2007;9(2):97.
23. Eliason S. Murder-suicide: a review of the recent literature. J Am Acad Psychiatry Law Online. 2009;37(3):371–6.
24. Tucker JM. Police officer willingness to use stress intervention services: the role of perceived organizational support (POS), confidentiality and stigma. Int J Emerg Mental Health Human Resilience. 2015;17(1):304.

5 Domestic Violence and the African American Community

Kathy C. Scott-Gurnell and Rahn Kennedy Bailey

Intimate partner violence (IPV), more often known as domestic violence, is a major public health problem and can only be dealt with in a multifactorial approach. Researchers continue to explore why African Americans have the highest incidence of domestic violence when compared to other races. Nearly one in four women and approximately one in seven men experience domestic partner abuse severe enough to be reported in their lifetime [1]. In a national representative survey conducted in 1996, 29% of African American women and 12% of African American men reported at least one instance of violence from an intimate partner [2]. In a more recent study in 2007, approximately 45% of Black women reported rape, physical violence, and stalking compared to 35% of the white population. When domestic partner violence gets extreme, this can lead to femicide (the killing of a woman) which is more common in African American women compared to whites [3]. Domestic violence has been known to lead to psychiatric issues such as depression, anxiety attacks, chronic depression, post-traumatic stress disorder, and suicidal ideation [4].

Cultural attitude and norms have been known to affect the reporting of IPV [5] within the African American population. This may lead to underreporting due to a belief in keeping the family unit together rather than exposing it. The coping mechanisms of IPV in Blacks (which include individuals of African and Caribbean descent) have been looked at in different studies. Cultural values of African Americans are known to affect how they cope and deal with IPV. Some do not attribute shoving and verbal abuse as domestic abuse and are able to tolerate more of this aggressive attitude from their partner. The culture of "protect the family" often prevents many women from sharing abuse. IPV is an important health issue in

K. C. Scott-Gurnell
Child & Adolescent Psychiatrist, Pearland, TX, USA

R. K. Bailey (✉)
Department of Psychiatry, Charles R. Drew University of Medicine and Science, Los Angeles, CA, USA
e-mail: rahnkbaileymd@comcast.net

R. K. Bailey (ed.), *Intimate Partner Violence*,
https://doi.org/10.1007/978-3-030-55864-2_5

African American women that needs special attention due to the underreporting of such cases. This highlights the importance of examining the role of culture when attempting to aid victims of abuse [6]. Lives may depend on it, especially since the mortality due to domestic violence in African American women is double that in white American women [7].

Substance abuse (alcohol, marijuana, and cocaine abuse) has been known to occur in relationships that involve IPV [8]. This is thought to be a reason why IPV is common in this group, although other factors experienced by many African Americans such as poverty and low socioeconomic status may aggravate partner abuse. A study done on the relationship between marijuana use and IPV in a national sample including whites, African Americans, Hispanics, Asian, and Native Americans found that abuse of marijuana during early adulthood and adolescent increases the risk of IPV [8].

> Religious activities such as attending churches and marriage counseling have positively impacted the growing crisis of domestic abuse in African Americans. Religious groups have supported the black community with education, fostering of young kids, and mentoring programs. Active participation in religion is one factor known to reduce the IPV in the African American population. The religion most African Americans practice is Christianity. This often involves going to church, hearing sermons from the Bible, and other educative sessions which can benefit couple's relationships. This may lead to better coping skills, allowing them deal with conflicts better without leading to IPV. Attending regular religious services is known to reduce the prevalence of IPV more so in African Americans, as well as to reduce substance abuse and mental health disorders [9].

Another contributing factor to increased incidence of violence displayed by African American men is institutional racism [10]. Black men may be frustrated with the way they are being treated by law enforcement agencies and authority figures. They also find difficulty in seeking jobs, which ultimately affects their income and financial potential. These external stressors may burden African American men and trigger violence with their spouses.

A study done examining adolescent females found some significant predictors that can influence the prevalence of dating violence in African American adolescents [10]. The study found one of the predictors included not knowing what a healthy relationship looks like. Some adolescents attribute physical, verbal, and other threats as a sign of love. This often leads to underreporting of partner violence. Other factors that can lead to adolescent females being vulnerable to dating violence from their respective male partner include watching porn videos and X-rated movies, drug use, and smoking marijuana. The study found an association between these predictors and dating partner violence.

Mental health disorders that have been linked to IPV include depression, anxiety, post-traumatic stress disorder, somatization disorder, suicidal ideations, and substance abuse [11].

How African Americans seek help when they are being abused may vary with the type of abuse they experience. Women who experience physical abuse also experience other types of abuse such as psychological, stalking, and sexual abuse [12]. A woman who has been sexually assaulted by her partner is less likely to report this finding because she may dread the blame would be put on her. Conversely, if assaulted by a stranger, she is more likely to seek help. Feelings of suffering psychologically in an abusive relationship are likely to be reported in African Americans [12].

African American women seek less help with an abusive partner due to fear of divorce and the stigma that goes along with it. Protecting the family can cause them to endure abuse. Most African Americans are in the lower socioeconomic class strata, thus having less funds and little time away from work, which can be a barrier to seeking medical and legal aid. Outpatient mental health services are not being used by African Americans as compared to the white population. However, African Americans are more likely to dial the police for help when they are experiencing severe abuse from their partner. The study identified the different types of abuse and how frequently they were being reported. In African Americans, stalking was reported the most. Stalking was more likely to lead individuals to seek help from sources such as family, friends, medical or mental health providers, police, and order of protection compared to ones who were physically abused alone. Individuals suffering from mostly sexual abuse obtained less help generally. African American women tend to report to more informal sources such as friends and churches than they do with more formal sources such as hospitals or legal institutions [13]. More educated women usually sought more help from a larger pool of resources. African American women were more likely to seek an order of protection compared to white women. The study found that health professionals were the resource used least in the reporting of domestic violence in African Americans. Approximately half of the African American women in this study developed symptoms of depression, which was not significantly related to seeking help or accessing resources.

In conclusion, cultural competency and sensitivity appear essential to assist African Americans experiencing IPV. The lack of understanding could greatly affect the ability to make a positive impact on the lives of African American men and women experiencing IPV.

References

1. CDC.gov. 2019. https://www.cdc.gov/violenceprevention/pdf/ipv-factsheet.pdf.
2. LaRen M. Domestic violence & black women. Blackdoctor. 2019 [cited 21 July 2019]. Available from: https://blackdoctor.org/13338/domestic-violence-signs-statistics-black-women__trashed/.
3. Lucea MB, Stockman JK, Mana-Ay M, Bertrand D, Callwood GB, Coverston CR, Campbell DW, Campbell JC. Factors influencing resource use by African American and African Caribbean women disclosing intimate partner violence. J Interpersonal Violence. 2013;28(8):1617–41.
4. Bent-Goodley TB. Perceptions of domestic violence: a dialogue with African American women. Health Social Work. 2004;29(4):307–16.
5. Stockman JK, Lucea MB, Bolyard R, Bertand D, Callwood GB, Sharps PW, Campbell DW, Campbell JC. Intimate partner violence among African American and African Caribbean women: prevalence, risk factors, and the influence of cultural attitudes. Glob Health Action. 2014;7(1):24772.
6. Lacey KK, Sears KP, Matusko N, Jackson JS. Severe physical violence and black women's health and well-being. Am J Public Health. 2015;105(4):719–24.

7. Long RA. Margaret webster plass: 1896–1990. African Arts. 1993;26(2):91–2.
8. Reingle JM, Staras SA, Jennings WG, Branchini J, Maldonado-Molina MM. The relationship between marijuana use and intimate partner violence in a nationally representative, longitudinal sample. J Interpersonal Violence. 2012;27(8):1562–78.
9. Ellison CG, Trinitapoli JA, Anderson KL, Johnson BR. Race/ethnicity, religious involvement, and domestic violence. Violence Against Women. 2007;13(11):1094–112.
10. Hampton R, Oliver W, Magarian L. Domestic violence in the African American community: an analysis of social and structural factors. Violence Against Women. 2003;9(5):533–57.
11. Follingstad DR. The impact of psychological aggression on women's mental health and behavior: the status of the field. Trauma Violence Abuse. 2009;10(3):271–89.
12. Flicker SM, Cerulli C, Zhao X, Tang W, Watts A, Xia Y, Talbot NL. Concomitant forms of abuse and help-seeking behavior among White, African American, and Latina women who experience intimate partner violence. Violence Against Women. 2011;17(8):1067–85.
13. Raiford JL, Wingood GM, DiClemente RJ. Prevalence, incidence, and predictors of dating violence: a longitudinal study of African American female adolescents. J Women's Health. 2007;16(6):822–32.

Intimate Partner Violence in Hispanic Communities

6

Ludmila De Faria

Intimate partner violence (IPV) disproportionally affects minorities [1]. In the United States, the Centers for Disease Control (CDC) estimates that about one in four women experience IPV [2].

According to the CDC "National Intimate Partner and Sexual Violence Survey (NISVS) 2010–2012" report, Hispanic women experience prevalence rate of violence similar to white women (34.4% vs 37.3%) [2].

Data for Hispanic women has been historically inconsistent [3, 4]. This rate may not be accurate for multiple reasons, most notably underreporting and underrepresentation in study populations [5].

Part of the issue with studying Hispanic populations in the United States comes from defining the population. Hispanic or Latino(a) is a term that refers to any Spanish culture or origin, regardless of race. This oversimplifies the cultural diversity within the population and conflates them into a homogenous block. In reality, Hispanic or Latino populations in the United States encompass groups as distinct as foreign-born and US-born; naturalized, undocumented, and permanent residents; and people from four different continents (North America, Central America, South America, and Europe). Lack of attention to the cultural diversity of this population and their unique perception of IPV may complicate the collection of data. Furthermore, high intermarriage rates and declining immigration are changing how Americans with Hispanic ancestry see their identity. About 11% of them do not self-identify as Hispanic, and that rate increases across generations [6].

Nevertheless, domestic violence and IPV are highly prevalent among Hispanic American populations, with two thirds of the female population (66.2%) experiencing more than one episode of victimization in their lifetime, 33.9% admitting to physical violence, 20.9% reporting sexual coercion, and 82.5% disclosing psychological aggression [7, 8]. Again, these rates may be inaccurate due to underreporting

L. De Faria (✉)
Department of Psychiatry, University of Florida College of Medicine, Gainesville, FL, USA
e-mail: l.barbosadefaria@ufl.edu

R. K. Bailey (ed.), *Intimate Partner Violence*,
https://doi.org/10.1007/978-3-030-55864-2_6

among unauthorized Hispanic immigrants [8]. Most of the data available rely on self-reporting or in data collected without culturally appropriate instruments or personnel [9]. Research efforts to obtain current numbers and develop interventions have been chronically hampered by the lack of appropriate sampling, and very few studies even try to include enough subjects from different subgroups [8, 10]. Current immigration policies have caused undocumented populations to avoid interfacing with authorities to report IPV for fear of deportation [11]. Lastly, perhaps the greatest barrier for abused immigrant women is language [12].

Disclosure of existing IPV when interfacing with medical, legal, or social services is only possible if Hispanic women have access to either staff who can speak their language or access to trained interpreters, via language lines provided by hospital or clinic. Lack of an appropriately trained and culturally competent interpreter may frustrate and discourage women from seeking and continuing services. Training staff on IPV and how to interview suspected victims is important, as the process may take more than one visit. Staff who are not trained may allow the abuser to participate in the interview process, either as a translator or collateral informant, increasing risk for the victim or silencing them [12]. On the other hand, the use of untrained interpreters may backfire. Interpreters may have poor boundaries, align with the abuser, or provide biased-based advice in the form of "counseling," re-traumatizing victims [13].

Vulnerable populations, including those from low socioeconomic status, may be at higher risk. The multiple disadvantage model holds that, when individuals are constrained by socioeconomic disadvantages, their social and intimate relationships can manifest the distress created by those disadvantages [14].

Last, but not least, lack of access to insurance remains a major barrier for women seeking help for IPV. Data indicates that 32% of women who visit an emergency room or seek help because of IPV tend to be either uninsured or to use Medicaid, as opposed to private insurance [14].

Other risk factors for Latinas are being married, number of ex-partners, diagnosis of depressions, disclosure of IPV to friends/family, mental health professionals, substance use, and partner's frequent alcohol use [14]. Women receiving negative social responses on disclosing their IPV may tend to experience more physical assaults than women receiving positive social responses, suggesting some abused women may perceive IPV as acceptable [14]. Access to culturally sensitive providers, who understand both culture and family dynamic and can respond appropriately to women when they chose to disclose, can facilitate help-seeking behavior.

Marriage and family are central to group-oriented cultures such as Hispanic and Latino, and traditional gender roles predominate. Within Latino culture, family includes not only immediate family but extended family and anyone else related to as family [15]. Hispanic cultural constructs of familismo, machismo, and marianismo illustrate well the role of culture. The idea of familismo encompasses family relations, loyalty, reciprocity, and solidarity [16]. The idea of family as the center that holds it all together is often reinforced by the elders in a multigenerational home, perpetuating the status quo and preventing women from seeking help by insisting on traditional gender roles. Women who break the silence and report the abuse may be criticized and isolated by the family and community at large. In addition to that, it is not uncommon for women to report that abuse has been perpetrated by multiple members of the family (in laws). In group-oriented cultures, where the needs of the community trample the needs of the individual, intergenerational trauma may also play a significant role in IPV. It is important to keep this in mind when conceptualizing and developing interventions for IPV in Hispanic populations. Furthermore, acculturation means different things for men and women, and both assimilation and acculturation are associated with greater risk for IPV, depending on context.

Machismo illustrates the role men play as the head of the household, the main provider, and decision-maker, displaying power through exaggerated sexual prowess and promiscuity [15]. The immigrant experience by itself can threaten a men's ability to fulfil his role due to unemployment and discrimination [17], increasing financial stressors and loss of their identity as providers. Marianismo, on the other hand, calls for women to self-sacrifice to maintain family integrity [18]. Many Hispanic women stay in an abusive relationship to prevent disintegration of family. On the other hand, women will leave an abusive relationship if they perceive that the family, especially children, are in danger [19]. The immigration process alters both men's and women's experiences [16, 20]. Less acculturated men hold on to this traditional role and may resent if their wives or girlfriends appear more independent (or more acculturated), increasing risk for IPV. Risk differs for different subgroups, likely reflecting how each ethnicity is treated and mainstreamed into American culture [20]. More acculturated or "Anglo-oriented" Latinas are more likely to talk about IPV and seek help. This opposes cultural norms in Hispanic communities [20] and increases risk for all types of victimization by exposing women to discrimination within their communities and loss of social support [20].

In conclusion, cultural constructs may influence the occurrence of IPV in the Hispanic/Latino community. Family are often the first individuals we turn to when seeking guidance and aid. Many cultures may minimize the seriousness of IPV. This is particularly true in patriarchal societies. Understanding the family dynamic can be exceedingly important in aiding victims of abuse. Hispanic individuals may have added challenges such as fear of deportation, language difficulty, and social isolation. All of these issues should be considered when attempting to understand victims of IPV who are within the Hispanic community.

References

1. Stockman JK, Hayashi H, Campbell JC. Intimate partner violence and its health impact on ethnic minority women. J Women's Health. 2015;24(1):62–79.
2. CDC. https://www.cdc.gov/violenceprevention/pdf/NISVS-StateReportBook.pdf. Accessed Dec 2017.
3. Tjaden PG, Thoennes N. Extent, nature, and consequences of intimate partner violence. National Institute of Justice. Findings from the National Violence Against Women Survey. 2000.
4. Cavanaugh CE, Messing JT, Amanor-Boadu Y, O'Sullivan CS, Webster D, Campbell J. Intimate partner sexual violence: a comparison of foreign-versus US-born physically abused Latinas. J Urban Health. 2014;91(1):122–35.

5. Montalvo-Liendo N. Cross-cultural factors in disclosure of intimate partner violence: an integrated review. J Adv Nurs. 2009;65(1):20–34.
6. Vidales GT. Arrested justice: the multifaceted plight of immigrant Latinas who faced domestic violence. J Family Violence. 2010;25(6):533–44.
7. Sawin EM, Sobel LL, Annan SL, Schminkey DL. From systematic review to call for action: in search of evidence-based interventions to decrease intimate partner violence in rural Hispanic American women. Hispanic Health Care Int. 2017;15(2):79–87.
8. Ogbonnaya IN, Finno-Velasquez M, Kohl PL. Domestic violence and immigration status among Latina mothers in the child welfare system: findings from the National Survey of Child and Adolescent Well-being II (NSCAW II). Child Abuse Negl. 2015;39:197–206.
9. Choi YJ, Elkins J, Disney L. A literature review of intimate partner violence among immigrant populations: engaging the faith community. Aggression Violent Behav. 2016;29:1–9.
10. Amerson R, Whittington R, Duggan L. Intimate partner violence affecting Latina women and their children. J Emerg Nursing. 2014;40(6):531–6.
11. Earner I. Double risk: immigrant mothers, domestic violence and public child welfare services in New York City. Evaluation Program Planning. 2010;33(3):288–93.
12. Stewart DE, Vigod S, Riazantseva E. New developments in intimate partner violence and management of its mental health sequelae. Curr Psychiatry Rep. 2016;18(1):4.
13. Alaggia R, Maiter S, Jenney A. In whose words? Struggles and strategies of service providers working with immigrant clients with limited language abilities in the violence against women sector and child protection services. Child Family Social Work. 2017;22(1):472–81.
14. Cheng TC, Lo CC. Racial disparities in intimate partner violence examined through the multiple disadvantage model. J Interpers Violence. 2016;31(11):2026–51.
15. Weidel JJ, Provencio-Vasquez E, Watson SD, Gonzalez-Guarda R. Cultural considerations for intimate partner violence and HIV risk in Hispanics. J Assoc Nurses AIDS Care. 2008;19(4):247–51.
16. Marin G, Marin BV. Research with Hispanic populations. Newbury Park: Sage; 1991.
17. Mancera BM, Dorgo S, Provencio-Vasquez E. Risk factors for Hispanic male intimate partner violence perpetration. Am J Mens Health. 2017;11(4):969–83.
18. Vazquez CI. The influence of gender role ideologies in women's careers: a look at Marianismo and machismo in the treatment room. IAFOR J Cult Stud. 2016;1(1) https://doi.org/10.22492/ijcs.1.1.02.
19. Kelly UA. "I'm a mother first": the influence of mothering in the decision-making processes of battered immigrant Latino women. Res Nurs Health. 2009;32(3):286–97.
20. Sabina C, Cuevas CA, Schally JL. The influence of ethnic group variation on victimization and help seeking among Latino women. Cult Divers Ethn Minor Psychol. 2015;21(1):19.

Intimate Partner Violence Among Muslim Immigrant Communities

7

Ulrick Vieux and Rahn Kennedy Bailey

> "The best among you is the one who treats his family the best, and I am the one who treats his family the best." (Prophet Muhammad)

Studies have shown that an estimated 4000 men murder their partners each year [1]. Approximately 1.5 million women are the victims of physical or sexual assault by intimate partners (IPV) each year [1]. Worldwide, an estimated 30% of women experience IPV during their lifetime, signaling that IPV is a widespread, costly problem [2]. In the United States, IPV affects a variety of individuals across many demographics. Traditionally, our impressions of IPV are often limited to husbands physically assaulting their wives during frequent domestic squabbles. We imagine these attacks to be spurred by financial difficulties, substance use, or the abject need of one partner to demonstrate power or control over the other. The reality is that IPV is not limited to race, creed, socioeconomic status, or gender. As providers, we must be cognizant of the variety of ways IPV can manifest. We must learn to expand and adapt our views of IPV beyond our narrow perceptions. As providers, in our interactions with our patients and clients, it is imperative for us to recognize various cultural nuances that may help us better identify IPV, as it occurs in various patient populations. To do this, we must first understand the nature of the problem, the ways in which it manifests in different populations, and the treatment barriers these populations face.

U. Vieux
Chairman and Psychiatry Residency Program Director at Garnet Health Medical Center, Middletown, NY, USA

R. K. Bailey (✉)
Department of Psychiatry, Charles R. Drew University of Medicine and Science, Los Angeles, CA, USA
e-mail: rahnkbaileymd@comcast.net

R. K. Bailey (ed.), *Intimate Partner Violence*,
https://doi.org/10.1007/978-3-030-55864-2_7

Vaughn et al. examined the prevalence of IPV in immigrant populations versus native-born Americans [3]. The researchers acknowledge that although immigrant populations are less likely to engage in criminal behavior than native-born Americans, IPV occurs more frequently within immigrant populations due to cultural norms that endorse patriarchal values. This accepted patriarchal hierarchy in immigrant communities legitimizes physical violence toward women by male aggressors [3]. Vaughn et al. found that immigrants were more likely to use physical violence against their spouses to the point of needing medical attention. Also, sexual violence was highly prevalent among these populations [3]. Additionally, Vaughn et al. assert, "In terms of lifetime victimization, however, immigrants were significantly less likely to report having been physically attacked, beaten, or injured by a spouse/partner" [3]. Immigrants from Latin America had the highest prevalence of IPV, followed by those from Asian, African, and European countries [3]. Vaughn et al. have enumerated a variety of reasons explaining why IPV is more prevalent among immigrant populations, chief of these being *acculturative stress* [3].

Acculturation refers to the idea that immigrant populations maintain their cultural identity despite relocating to the United States. The struggle for immigrant populations is in reconciling their cultural beliefs to fit Western ideals. Oftentimes, immigrants take solace in preserving their cultural identities in foreign, unknown settings. The cultural framework deemed acceptable in other cultures may not translate into their new surroundings, and relocating a family of non-native English speakers to the U.S. is fraught with challenges. Gupta et al. examined the link between non-native English speakers, length of time in the United States, and incidence of IPV. They found that non-recent immigrant men with limited English-speaking acuity were at the highest risk of IPV perpetration [4]. Further, Gupta concedes that although IPV perpetration among recent immigrant men was lower when compared to nonimmigrants, the reverse is true for settled immigrants who have spent more time in the United States [4]. This inverse relationship between time spent in the United States and lack of fluency in English demonstrates the idea of acculturative stress. Despite spending long periods of time in the United States, certain immigrant communities are reticent to even combat language barriers, much less culturally adhere to Western traditions or mores. Further, men are usually the primary breadwinners in the household due to work visa constraints, educational disparities, and cultural constraints regarding women in the workforce. Oftentimes, women household members are left completely dependent on the primary earner for survival. Thus, they tend to experience social isolation compounded by their own language barriers and tenuous immigration status. These women often have no recourse but to stick with their partners despite the presence of IPV in the household.

The growing and vibrant immigrant Muslim community, like many other communities, has had to deal with the scourge of intimate partner violence. Within the Muslim community, a significant diversity exists among native-born and immigrant-born Muslims. This diversity is manifested along lines of ethnicity, race, socioeconomic status, level of education, and interpretation of Islamic scripture. Specific challenges relevant to the immigrant Muslim community are the following [5]:

1. Isolation – Relocation to a new country in which the language, food, culture, and weather are all foreign leads to stress. In addition, if Islamophobia is prevalent, this will lead to further isolation. Abusers will take full advantage of the victim's vulnerable position.
2. Stigma – Shame and embarrassment are emotions that victims of IPV may constantly carry. Compounded with these feelings is the perceived shame that disclosing abuse can be used to disgrace family and community.
3. Discrimination – Trust is essential in order to build the therapeutic alliance that is required to address IPV. Communities that are ostracized by mainstream society and demonized by politicians will have difficulty confiding and believing in secular authorities with their intimate family dynamics.
4. Community pressure – Divorce and separation are allowed in Islam, even though they are not ideal. Divorce can be viewed as a stigmatizing event, even if necessary. As a result, members of the victim's family and community can discourage victims from making decisions that might be in their best interest.
5. Lack of knowledge of rights within Islam – There may be assumptions that a person culturally identifying as Muslim understands the empathic nuances of the faith, as revealed by Prophet Muhammad and his Ahlul-Bayt (progeny). As a result, cultural practices that are an anathema to Islam, such as honor killings and genital mutilation, may be condoned by the culture.
6. Immigration status vulnerability – The threat of deportation can hinder victims from advocating for themselves.
7. Fear of losing custody of children or child abduction – The threat of losing their children is often used to intimidate victims.

The issue of IPV has well-documented mental health, reproductive health, and chronic physical health consequences [2]. Muslim clerics, like many clerics of different faiths, may not have the necessary skills to effectively deal with victims of IPV; yet, they will often be the first person consulted in these issues. Hence, the importance of providing education for clerics and establishing collaborative relationships between mental health professionals and clerics cannot be overemphasized.

Case Study

Zainab is a 21-year-old Hispanic female, Muslim convert who presents to the outpatient mental health clinic. She presents with anxiety, depression, and symptoms of post-traumatic stress disorder after experiencing the disillusionment and dissolution of her religious marriage and tumultuous 2-year relationship to Omar, a 26-year-old first-generation immigrant male from a predominantly Muslim country. Zainab was raised a Catholic and converted to Islam at the age of 18 when she was a freshman in college. She is a nurse by profession and met Omar while in college, when he was a pre-med student.

Zainab changed her name after converting to Islam, and she was raised in a working-class neighborhood in New York City. She reported being active in a neighborhood church growing up and attended a Catholic high school where her parents struggled to pay her tuition. While at college she was intrigued by the diversity of her classmates. Her attraction to Islam first started after befriending African-American and Arab Muslim classmates in an introductory biology class. She befriended several Muslim students and subsequently joined the MSA (Muslim Student Association) in her school. Zainab expressed empathy toward the Muslim community, and the history of Islam resonated with her, especially the story of her namesake, Zainab, the granddaughter of Prophet Muhammad, and her role in the historical event of Karbala.

Zainab felt fortunate when compared to many converts in that her parents were supportive of her conversion to Islam – a constant source of support. During this time she met Omar, the son of professionals, grew up in the middle to upper class suburb of New York City, and his parents immigrated to the United States in the 1970s. His parents were very active and helped fund the mosque in his community. The mosque that Omar grew familiar with was homogenous and catered mostly to the people of his community, something not unique to many of the mosques that he was accustomed to in his area of the country. The Muslim cleric that led this mosque was originally from the country that the founders of the mosque immigrated. English was the clerics second language, and he was not completely comfortable living in the United States.

Similar to Zainab, Omar found college to be an invigorating experience. He found college and his subsequent membership in the MSA to be an opportunity for learning about the faith of his cultural heritage. Admittedly, Omar was not overtly religious, as he drank alcohol, engaged in premarital sex, and was ambivalent about performing the five daily prayers, for example. However, he was very politically involved in international Muslim affairs, specifically as it concerned the Middle East. The MSA afforded him an opportunity to meet other Muslims of different backgrounds, and this provided him an opportunity to further understand his faith. However, certain cultural issues negatively impacted him, and unaddressed mental health issues stymied him.

Omar was intrigued by Zainab, and a friendship was established. As a convert to Islam, Zainab found Omar's background in Islam fascinating. She was impressed by his ability to read the Quran in Arabic and the number of chapters (sura) he had committed to memory. Omar was impressed by Zainab's passion of the deen and her desire to apply many of the lessons found in Quran and Hadith. As their relationship blossomed, and in order to ensure that their relationship remained within the guidelines of Islam, both felt it was essential to have a Muslim marriage. The marriage was attended by close friends on campus, though it was not legally recognized. Omar did not feel comfortable telling his parents about the relationship, knowing and understanding that his parents and family would not approve of a marriage with someone not of their culture. The lack of support and Omar's ambivalence led to significant stress in the relationship. Zainab continued to develop in the understanding of her faith and rights, and as a result, Omar became intimidated and threatened by her growth. During this time Omar's parents were actively looking at possible spouses for Omar. Unfortunately, in addition to becoming verbally abusive to Zainab, he also became physically abusive. Eventually, with the support of her friends and the college cleric, Zainab decided to request an Islamic divorce from Omar. As a result, Zainab presents to the student mental health clinic on campus to receive counseling for her current feelings of hopelessness and difficulty with trust.

Key Points of Discussion

"Marriage is a partnership based on love and mercy." (Quran 30: 21)

The Muslim community in the United States is a vibrant community that has contributed immensely to the American fabric. From enslaved Africans, who laid the economic fabric for the success of the country, to current immigrants from places such as Somalia, the contribution is significant. In addition, the American Muslim community is diverse in multiple areas ranging from race, ethnicity, education, and socioeconomic status. Faith is an essential aspect of the day-to-day lives of Muslims. For example, according to a 2017 Pew Research Center survey, within the African-American community, a majority of both Black Muslims (75%) and Black Christians (84%) reported that religion is very important to them [6]. However, even though one in five American Muslim adults were raised in a different faith tradition and converted to Islam, a similar percentage of Americans who were raised Muslim now no longer identify with the faith [7]. Fifty-eight percent of US Muslim adults come from another part of the world, and their presence is due to the civil rights movement of the 1960s. Specifically due to the 1965 Immigration and Nationality Act that lowered barriers to immigration from Asia, Africa, and other regions outside of Europe [8]. A key similarity between immigrants and US-born Muslims is that religious practice is similar. The key difference is that immigrants tend to come from a higher socioeconomic background [8]. It is estimated that there are 3–4.5 million Muslims of all ages living in the United States as of 2017 [7]. According to the Institute for Social Policy, "American Muslims are the only faith community surveyed with no majority race, with 25% black, 24% white, 18% Asian, 18% Arab, 7% mixed race, and 5% Hispanic" [9]. As a result of this diversity, many of the problems that are seen in society as a whole will also be seen within the Muslim community.

Domestic violence is a scourge that affects people across all lines of race, age, ethnicity, socioeconomic status, and religion. According to the Centers for Disease Control and Prevention, one out of four women are victims of severe domestic violence. Therefore, it is problematic to solely paint domestic violence as a problem unique to the Muslim community. However, due to Islamophobia and the sad reality that some Muslims do not understand their religion – the Muslim victim of domestic violence is especially vulnerable. For example, according to the Institute for Social Policy and Understanding, domestic violence equally plagues most faith communities. In addition, the Muslim community is more likely to report domestic violence to faith leaders. This signifies the importance of educating and providing social services to the victims of domestic violence. Shelters provide an enormous resource for victims of domestic violence who are seeking shelter from their tormentors and may not have the resources. The staff provides empathy for their Muslim clients. Examples of suboptimal shelters could be victims being subject to Islamophobic statements from staff and not having access to halal meals.

Peaceful Families Project (PFP) is an organization taking the lead in addressing this problem by providing cultural sensitivity trainings and technical assistance for professionals, conducting research, and developing resources. Such projects help provide the support that is needed to help these survivors help themselves.

References

1. Kulwicki A, Ballout S, Kilgore C, Hammad A, Dervartanian H. Intimate partner violence, depression, and barriers to service utilization in Arab American women. J Transcult Nurs. 2015;26(1):24–30.
2. Hawcroft C, Hughes R, Shaheen A, Usta J, Elkadi H, Dalton T, et al. Prevalence and health outcomes of domestic violence among clinical populations in Arab countries: a systemic review and meta-analysis. BMC Public Health. 2019;19:315.
3. Vaughn MG, Salas-Wright CP, Cooper-Sadlo S, Maynard BR, Larson M. Are immigrants more likely than native-born Americans to perpetrate intimate partner violence? J Interpers Violence. 2015;30(11):1888–904.
4. Gennadi M, Giuliani C, Accordini M. Muslim immigrants men's and women's attitudes toward intimate partner violence. Eur J Psychol. 2017;13(4):688–707.
5. Fontes LA. Immigrant Muslim couples and domestic violence. Psychology Today. 2017.
6. Mohamed B, Diamant J. Black Muslims account for a fifth of all U.S. Muslims, and about half are converts to Islam. Pew Research Center. January 17, 2019. https://www.pewresearch.org/fact-tank/2019/01/17/black-muslims-account-for-a-fifth-of-all-u-s-muslims-and-about-half-are-converts-to-islam/.
7. Mohamed B. New estimates show U.S. Muslim population continues to grow. Pew Research Center. January 3, 2018. https://www.pewresearch.org/fact-tank/2018/01/03/new-estimates-show-u-s-muslim-population-continues-to-grow/.
8. Muslims in America: immigrants and those born in U.S. see life differently in many ways. April 17, 2018. https://pewforum.org/essay/muslims-in-america-immigrants-and-those-born-in-u-s-see-life-differently-in-many-ways/.
9. American Muslim Poll 2017: Key Findings|ISPU. https://www.ispu.org/american-muslim-poll-2017-key-findings/. Institute for social policy and understanding. March 21, 2017. Retrieved November 23, 2019.

8 Same-Sex Partner Violence: A Look at Domestic Violence in the LGBTQ Community

Mark H. Townsend and Rahn Kennedy Bailey

Although intimate partner violence (IPV) is increasingly recognized as a public health emergency, violence between same-sex partners is less understood and more easily ignored. Indeed, those responding to the acute effects of violence between or against members of sexual minority communities may bring unhelpful, even dangerous preconceptions to their work. Some may incorrectly believe that lesbian, gay, bisexual, transgender, and queer/questioning (LGBTQ) couples are less violent. Others may assume that same-sex couples have less power inequity than between heterosexual partners [1]. A study using the 2005–2007 Behavioral Risk Factor Surveillance System (BRFSS) date to compare IPV in opposite and same-sex relationships found few differences in the types of domestic violence experienced, despite fewer services for same-sex IPV victims [2]. Men and women were as likely to experience physical and sexual abuse by male partners as by female; women in same-sex relationships were also more likely to experience verbal abuse.

Though both same-sex and opposite-sex couples experience and report IPV, care must be taken to understand the unique issues that affect same-sex relationships. A number of factors, including prevailing gender roles, societal expectations, and stigma, can make addressing intimate partner violence among same-sex couples challenging. It should be stated that same-sex couples are affected by factors such as discrepancies in age, socioeconomic status, and race that place stress on most relationships. This may play into the power dynamics within a couple.

Heterosexism describes the discrimination against LGBTQ individuals founded on the belief that heterosexuality is correct/normal/superior [3]. This, along with

M. H. Townsend
George C Dunn Professor of Psychiatry, Louisiana State University Health Sciences Center New Orleans, New Orleans, LA, USA

R. K. Bailey (✉)
Department of Psychiatry, Charles R. Drew University of Medicine and Science, Los Angeles, CA, USA
e-mail: rahnkbaileymd@comcast.net

R. K. Bailey (ed.), *Intimate Partner Violence*,
https://doi.org/10.1007/978-3-030-55864-2_8

fixed beliefs on gender roles, has created misconceptions about who can be both the perpetrator, as well as the victim of intimate partner abuse. These narrow viewpoints have largely shaped how society views intimate partner violence. Intimate partner violence, from a legal perspective, can be defined as "any assault, battery, sexual assault, sexual battery, or any criminal offense resulting in physical injury or death of one family or household member by another who is or was residing in the same dwelling" [4].

Although this seems to be a very broad and encompassing definition, misinformation largely predetermines how society thinks about intimate partner violence and domestic abuse. Many have accepted the common phenomenon of intimate partner violence. However, several misconceptions remain.

Common misconceptions are:

- Some people deserve it.
- If the nature of abuse is not physical, then it is not that serious.
- Most cases are simply brought upon by drinking or drugs.
- It is only a poor person's problem.
- If it is bad, a victim can just leave.
- All abuse is perpetrated by males against female partners [4].

These often prevalent misconceptions can have influence on those in advocacy and legal agencies. Additionally, it has been stated many times throughout this book that abusive partners have coercive control over their victims. This adds an additional complication if an abusive partner threatens to out their victims to friends, family, or employers [4]. Further still, an abuser may keep their victim isolated from the gay community. Naturally, this reduces the chance of disclosing abuse to an understanding and possibly helpful community. Moreover, a victim may be shamed into not reporting abuse. A perpetrator may say reporting abuse "will make the gay community look bad" [4]. Sadly, a victim may remain reticent in order to uphold the reputation of their community. Understanding these additional social burdens and dynamics is necessary to helping and understanding victims who may be in an untraditional relationship.

Homophobia and its impact on the lives of LGBTQ individuals have been increasingly researched. The term "minority stress" has been used to describe societal burdens that are experienced by a minority population. These burdens are often associated with low social status that is bestowed on socially disenfranchised people.

Brooks (1981) defines minority stress as "The cultural ascription of inferior status to particular groups. This ascription of defectiveness to various categories of people, particularly categories based on sex, race, and sociosexual preference, and precipitates negative life events...over which the individual has little or no control" [4, 5].

The effects of minority stress can be compounded. For example, a lesbian may endure more minority stress than a gay man. This is attributed to women often having lower social status. Furthermore, a lesbian of color would experience even more of a minority stress burden by virtue of being a woman, homosexual, and a racial minority, i.e., composed of all oppressed and disenfranchised entities [4].

It is important to note what some potential minority stress can arise from. Things such as hate, hate crimes, discrimination, homophobia, and the fear of being outed can all contribute to minority stress. This additional stress can cause turmoil in a same-sex relationship [4]. Studies have reported evidence that linked greater levels of minority stress with lower relationship quality and both intimate partner abuse perpetration and victimization [4]. So, it is important to consider the multitude of cultural, social, political, and religious stressors that may play into the mental and physical health of those in the gay, lesbian, and bi communities. Past experiences with stressors such as bigotry, discrimination, and hate can inform how a victim of abuse seeks (or does not seek) help. In order for an individual to disclose abuse, they must have sense of safety, security, and trust. In a homophobic society, it can be difficult (understandably so) for gay, lesbian, and bisexual individuals to trust that they will not be discriminated against. This is especially true if their lack of trust is in accordance with their own past experiences [4]. This makes the issue of minority stress an exceedingly important factor for one to consider when tackling the issue of intimate partner violence among gay, lesbian, and bisexual individuals.

Another equally important influence on gay, lesbian, and bisexual communities is society's overarching view on gender roles. This can create difficulty for people such as law enforcement to identify victim vs perpetrator. This is usually built on the preconception that the male is always the perpetrator and the female is always the victim [4]. This can leave some befuddled when they are confronted with intimate partner violence in a same-sex couple. Indeed, some may feel that individuals in a same-sex relationship are evenly matched (physically/socially). The view that same-sex partners are equal in power and status is coupled with the idea that males are naturally aggressive and females are more docile. This misconception is particularly counterproductive to understanding intimate partner violence among lesbian couples. Regarding lesbian couples, it is often assumed women are both nonviolent and equal to their partner. This notion is sometimes present in lesbian communities. This creates an "invisible" problem [4]. That is to say, due to decreased openness to the possibility of violence, victims may not disclose abuse. Sadly, some lesbian victims may blame themselves and feel as though they are the source of the problem [4].

Similarly, intimate partner violence has its own societal misconceptions. Particularly, the prevailing view is that a man cannot be the victim of domestic violence [4]. Additionally, there is some degree of acceptance that a certain degree of violence is normal among men. If the prevailing view is that only females are victims, many men may not report abuse for fear of being "feminized" [4]. Thus, they will often be left to endure abuse in isolation as well.

Most gay, lesbian, and bisexual individuals are raised in households with heterosexism and typical gender roles, creating an early idea of what is typical behavior for boys and girls. These views are often carried into and influence views on relationships later in life [4]. This leads to generalizations that all male/male relationships are violent and all female/female are not [4]. Not only is this view incorrect, but it leads one to believe that same-sex intimate partner violence is more trivial than that seen in heterosexual relationships.

A series of questionnaires given to 200 lesbians found that barriers to reporting abuse were fear of loss of confidentiality and lack of trust of service providers [4]. Sadly, some respondents went on to report that some shelters were unwelcoming and unsupportive. In this same questionnaire, an important factor was brought to light. Some women reported that they were not able to seek help from family members because they (family) did not know that they were lesbian/in a relationship [4].

Intimate partner violence can place victims at higher risk for STI including HIV [5].

Thus, creating groups of those in positions to help (shelters, health care, legal, and law enforcement) may be too inadequate or inexperienced to help [6].

Equal protection under the law has be a hard-fought goal for gay rights advocates. Regarding intimate partner violence protection, some have been hesitant to grant equal legal protection. Here is a noteworthy example: in 1994, a case involving court order protection and same-sex couples was brought to light. A Kentucky Court of Appeals ruled that orders of protection from domestic violence should be issued to same-sex couples [6]. As it was written, the law used gender neutral language. The law framed domestic violence as involving "any family member or member of an unmarried couple" [6].

Before the case was decided, Kentucky State Senator Tim Philpot proposed a revision to the law. Specifically, he desired to change the phrase of "an unmarried couple" to "individuals of the opposite sex," citing that the law was intended "to protect women and children from abuse and protect a traditional family unit" [6]. Later, the state legislature held hearings on the matter and ruled that any victim of violence is free to file criminal charges [6]. Incensed over this issues and gay marriage, State Senator Philpot famously quipped, "I do not agree that gay couples fit the definition of family. It hasn't happened in the history of the world" [6].

In February 2013, the Violence Against Women Act was reauthorized. In this rendition, the act uses language that specifically includes lesbians and transgender people.

These are important expansions that have occurred at the federal level. However, the majority of criminal cases involving domestic violence are conducted at the state level [7].

A large portion of state family law statutes pertain to obtaining orders of protection [7].

When considering seeking help, many victims are burdened with a sense of shame and the fear of judgment. This is doubly so for those who are in a same-sex relationship. This can lead to social isolation and helplessness unique to this population. In this society of heterosexuality as "normal," many individuals who are in same sex relationships may be closeted [7, 8]. If a homosexual relationship is abusive, there may be the added obstacle of not wanting to disclose sexuality that may keep some from seeking help [9]. This attitude may trivialize how serious intimate partner violence in gay, lesbian, and bisexual couples can be [10]. This makes understanding how gender role influence same-sex couples exceedingly important [10].

This lack of openness regarding same-sex relationships and the abuse therein has led to an attitude of diminished severity in the public eye. Likely, the downplaying of intimate partner violence among gay, lesbian, and bi communities was done to avoid negative publicity [11]. This was probably intended to protect against further discrimination. However, this may have detracted from the legal recognition of such unions [12].

In addition to limited legal protection, those in the gay, lesbian, bisexual community face a higher likelihood of being beaten in an act of anti-gay/homophobic violence [12]. Moreover, anti-gay organizations may use reports of domestic violence to reinforce their viewpoint that homosexuality or a homosexual relationship is inherently doomed, dangerous, flawed, and unsafe [12]. Transgender individuals may be subject to even higher rates of sexual violence, much of it characterized as IPV [13]. Transwomen of color may be among the most vulnerable, their status as members of two marginalized communities adversely affecting their ability to secure adequate housing and employment, thus facilitating situations conducive to IPV. For example, murder rates, and incidents of unnecessarily violent "over-kill" murders, have been reported to be higher among African-American transwomen [14]. Incarceration rates are not only thought to be higher among these women, but also upon incarceration, they are more likely to experience sexual assault [15].

Thus, many in the LGBTQ community are faced with a dilemma. Awareness and aid is needed to help those in abusive relationships. However, there is an inherent risk of negative publicity in bringing to light this aspect of same-sex relationships. This may be anathema to the positive image that same-sex relationships are now garnering in the media and pop culture. Indeed, some may have to wrestle with exposing this dark aspect of same-sex relationships or remain silent in hopes that the new-found acceptance and tolerance of same-sex relationships is preserved. Consolation may be found in the fact that intimate partner violence occurs at similar levels in both same-sex and heterosexual relationships [12].

Intimate partner violence among same-sex relationships is socially and legally complex. It has long been hidden in the gay community. Originally, it was not a focal point of the anti-domestic violence movement [12]. Interestingly, the occurrence of intimate partner violence in the context of same-sex relationships is vexing. This challenges some established feminist viewpoints. Specifically, the notion that domestic violence is gender-specific is brought into question [12]. Particularly, it has been emphasized among feminists that intimate partner violence is largely a male-evoked exertion of power and aggression [12]. This idea is challenged by female-to-female intimate partner violence that occurs. The first comprehensive study, the National Coalition of Anti-Violence Programs (1997), took an in-depth look at violence in same-sex communities. The study defined intimate partner violence as "verbal, physical, financial, and/or sexual abuse occurring in the context of a romantic relationship" [12]. Under this definition, the study found that approximately between 25% and 33% of same-sex relationships involve physical or psychological abuse [12]. Organizations that are anti-gay are often quick to cite an example(s) of domestic disharmony among same-sex relationships as proof of the ill-fated nature of such relationships. In the late 1990s, an edition of Culture Facts, a weekly periodical tied to the anti-gay organization, the Family Research Council, produced a damning story. The story was related to same-sex violence and appeared in a section entitled "'Gay' Violence Escalates." Therein it was reported that 47.5% of lesbians experience some form of domestic abuse compared with only 0.22% of married heterosexual women [12]. The current consensus is that these statistics were grossly exaggerated [12].

However, it does neatly fit into a popular anti-homosexual narrative that a homosexual individual "is their own worst enemy" [12]. The implication of this type of sentiment being that gay men bring HIV upon themselves and lesbians have to endure the increased risk of intimate partner violence (due to their lifestyle). For years, the prevailing method of attacking homosexuality has been to focus on male homosexuality. Male homosexuality has been described as "unnatural" and abnormal. Conversely, not much has be said about lesbian relationships (using such harsh terms) [12]. With the increased awareness of intimate partner violence among lesbian couples, some have used this a platform for advocating against such relationships.

Intimate partner violence has been shown to occur at the same rate among both homosexual and heterosexual relationships. Intimate partner violence in same-sex relationships is largely the same as in heterosexual relationships. The abuser typically exercises coercive control. Control is maintained by the use of physical violence, threats, verbal, and psychological abuse. Similarly, victims who are in same-sex relationships endure the same amount/type of suffering as their heterosexual counterparts [16]. Some of the sufferings endured are fear, anxiety, depression, physical injury, and even death [16]. This range was commensurate to the incidence of violence found in opposite-sex relationships. However according to the study invisible victims: same-sex IPV in the National Violence Against Women Survey, bisexual individuals were at the highest risk of being victimized by an opposite sex partner [17]. Bisexual women report domestic violence rates that are higher than those reported by either heterosexual or lesbian women [18]. 5.5% of women between the ages of 18 and 44 years identify as bisexual. This makes bisexual women the largest sexual minority group [19].

With greater public awareness, the number of reported intimate partner violence rates increases. In the year following the study released by the National Coalition of Anti-Violence Programs, the number of reported cases increased. A survey released in October 1998 shows a 41% nationwide increase in reported cases of same-sex domestic violence [20]. San Francisco saw a 67% increase in reported cases after the District Attorney Office took proactive measures. The office commissioned a victims' advocate with the explicit purpose to work with reported instances of same-sex intimate partner violence [20].

This bolsters the need to fight against homophobia to foster trust among those who may be hesitant to disclose their sexual orientation to those who could potentially offer help such as family, social workers, advocates, law enforcement, or the judicial system.

This is not the only reason that those in the gay, lesbian, and bisexual community may be reluctant to disclose or publicize intimate partner violence. The image of same-sex relationships as egalitarian and peaceful has been carefully crafted. Through years of mindfulness about public perception, society (both those in and outside of the homosexual community) has an expectation of harmony among same-sex individuals/relationship. Indeed, it can be hard to reconcile the notion that same-sex individuals deliberately hurt, threaten, batter, terrorize, stalk, and even kill one another.

In grappling with the idea that women in same-sex relationship commit intimate partner violence, some have highlighted concerns regarding the proper handling of violence. Rightly or wrongly, males are often presumed to be the aggressor during domestic violence investigations. In dealing with female/female intimate partner violence, such presumptions are not easily made [21]. This issue can be even less clear-cut with respect to women's shelters. Often the overarching policy is "to believe the woman." Often the question is posed "how does one determine which woman to believe?"

Archaic views on intimate partner violence do not precisely fit the narrative of same-sex intimate partner violence. Classic views on intimate partner violence stem from a patriarchal perspective. From this perspective, a man seeks to control a female. This is built on the historical status of women as property.

However, it must be reiterated that men can be victims and women can be perpetrators of abuse. Thus, we need to think of domestic violence as a multifaceted and complex phenomenon that occurs irrespective of gender, gender role, or biological sex. Likely, gender is one of many factors such as race, socioeconomic class, ability, and sexual orientation that influence power dominance dynamics.

Sexual orientation in particular becomes important if a victim is not "out" (openly gay). Threats can be levied against a victim threatening to expose their sexuality. Some individuals may be selective in whom they share their sexual identity with. For example, close friends may be made privy to one's homosexuality/bisexuality, while employers or family may be kept in the dark. This is like done to elude homophobia. Homophobia can be manifested as the loss of safety, emotional support, employment, or financial support.

This again brings to the forefront how homophobia plays into how a victim seeks help. Unlike in a heterosexual relationship, an individual in a same-sex relationship is more subject to bigotry in society. For someone in a same-sex relationship, disclosing their sexuality may be unavoidable when seeking help from law enforcement, shelters, or the courts. This subjects them to the possibility of additional judgment and discrimination. The fear of reinforcing misconceptions may keep those in the gay, lesbian, and bisexual community from disclosing abuse. This can be difficult regarding coming out to family members. Additionally, many in the LGBTQ community face the possibility of being victimized in a hate crime if they disclose their identity [21].

The threat of facing homophobia is present in shelters as well. Although a woman may not be outright denied access to a shelter, she can still experience discrimination and homophobia.

Indeed, some lesbians have reported feeling unwelcome at shelters. This is mainly attributed to the attitude of the other women who reside in the shelter. There may be concern regarding "sharing a sleeping space." To avoid this, some women refer to their abuser by a masculine pronoun. This can further isolate lesbian individuals. Sadly, it may even impede the healing process.

Shelters often are supported by government funding. If those in government have conservative or hold anti-gay views, this could prove problematic in securing funding. In this day-and-age, that scenario may seem ridiculous. However, it does have precedence. In the 1980s, Attorney General Edwin Meese wanted desperately to revoke a Justice Department grant to the National Coalition Against Domestic Violence because it was too "pro-lesbian" [6]. Sentiments like this can (understandably) create mistrust of law enforcement and those in the judicial system among LGBTQ individuals.

It is true, society has evolved to become more accepting of same-sex relationships. Thus more people have felt safer in disclosing their sexuality. Though the trend has moved toward social equality, it is important to note that many in the gay, lesbian, bisexual, and trans community still remain in close interconnected communities [22]. This means that often times the abuser and victim may have many mutual friends and associates.

Has the law evolved and expended to offer protections to same-sex intimate partner victims? The Violence Against Women Act was a law passed in 1994. The law originally offered protections for women in heterosexual relationships [23]. However, it has since been expanded to include more inclusive protections. The law allowed for domestic violence crimes to fall under federal jurisdiction. Additionally, it directed states to enforce protection orders issued by other jurisdictions [23].

California is particularly noteworthy for its requirements for obtaining protective orders. In California, criminal charges do not need to be filed against the respondent before a protective order can be issued [23]. California has a progressive approach in dealing with those who have been convicted in domestic violence battery. Batterers must complete a 1-year batterer's intervention treatment program [23].

State law on domestic violence varies widely on its inclusion of protections for gay, lesbian, and bisexual individuals. For example, Hawaii has some of the most inclusive state laws [23]. Conversely, Montana has a narrower stance on legal recourse to be offered to victims of domestic abuse. Under Montana's law, action is taken when an offense occurs with "bodily injury" to family members or "partners." "Partners," however, are "spouses, former spouses, [and] persons who have been or are currently in a dating or ongoing intimate relationship with a person of the opposite sex" [23].

In 2000, New York City had the largest community of same-sex couples [23]. However, in New York state (circa 2000), domestic violence was not considered a crime when committed against someone of the same sex (who is not a relative) [23]. New York's Family Court Act was amended in 2010 to include gender neutral language [23].

At the state level, there is no universal definition of an intimate partner violence victim. This leaves potential for many to still be neglected.

In conclusion, intimate partner violence occurs in relationships involving both same-sex and heterosexual couples. Over, the past 40 years, both society and the law have become cognizant of domestic violence. Indeed, much has been done to remedy and prevent the problem. However, most of the social and legal advances have benefited heterosexual women. Traditionally, women's shelters, advocacy centers, and law enforcement were attuned to the struggle this demographic endures (regarding domestic abuse). As time has passed, IPV has been seen as a phenomenon that affects a broader range of people. Though women are indeed abused by male partners, this is not the only flavor of intimate partner violence. In heterosexual relationships, females abuse males. Both males and females abuse each other in same-sex relationships. It is very laudable that through increased awareness, this fact has been brought to light. However, many in same-sex relationships are still reluctant to disclose abuse in their relationships. Fear of judgment and discrimination are the major reasons why. Sadly, close-minded and bigoted views on homosexuality still persist in society. Moreover, some of these antiquated views are still reflected in the law. At the state level, many vulnerable people still do not enjoy the fullest protection of the law.

References

1. Renzetti CM, Miley CH. Violence in gay and lesbian domestic partnerships [special issue]. J Gay Lesbian Soc Serv. 1996;4:1.
2. Blosnich JR, Bossarte RM. Comparisons of intimate partner violence among partners in same-sex and opposite-sex relationships in the United States. Am J Public Health. 2009;99(12):2182–4.
3. Krieger N. A glossary for social epidemiology. J Epidemiol Community Health. 2001;55:693–700.
4. Brown C. Gender-role implications on same-sex intimate partner abuse. J Family Violence. 2008;23(6):457–62.
5. Duncan DT, Goedel WC, Stults CB, Brady WJ, Brooks FA, Blakely JS, Hagen D. A study of intimate partner violence, substance abuse, and sexual risk behaviors among gay, bisexual, and other men who have sex with men in a sample of geosocial-networking smartphone application users. Am J Mens Health. 2018;12(2):292–301.
6. Letellier P. Gay and bisexual male domestic violence victimization: challenges to feminist theory and responses to violence. Violence Victims. 1994;9(2):95.
7. Burke LK, Follingstad DR. Violence in lesbian and gay relationships: theory, prevalence, and correlational factors. Clin Psychol Rev. 1999;19(5):487–512.
8. Greenwood GL, Relf MV, Huang B, Pollack LM, Canchola JA, Catania JA. Battering victimization among a probability-based sample of men who have sex with men. Am J Public Health. 2002;92(12):1964–9.
9. Ard KL, Makadon HJ. Addressing intimate partner violence in lesbian, gay, bisexual, and transgender patients. J General Int Med. 2011;26(8):930–3.
10. Alhusen JL, Lucea MB, Glass N. Perceptions of and experience with system responses to female same-sex intimate partner violence. Partn Abus. 2010;1(4):443.
11. Rollè L, Giardina G, Caldarera AM, Gerino E, Brustia P. When intimate partner violence meets same sex couples: a review of same sex intimate partner violence. Frontiers Psychol. 2018;9:1506.
12. Brooks VR. Minority stress and lesbian women. Lexington, MA. Lexington Books. Carter WC, Feld SL. Principles relating social regard to size and density of personal networks with applications to stigma. Social Networks. 1981;26:3232329.
13. Drescher CF, Griffin JA, Casanova FK, Wood E, Brands S, Stepleman LM. Associations of physical and sexual violence victimization, homelessness, and perceptions of safety with suicidality in a community sample of transgender individuals. Psychol Sexuality. 2019; https://doi.org/10.1080/19419899.2019.1690032.
14. Stotzer RL. Data sources hinder our understanding of transgender murders. Am J Public Health. 2017;107(9):1362–3.

15. Reisner SL, Bailey Z, Sevelius J. Racial/ethnic disparities in history of incarceration, experiences of victimization, and associated health indicators among ransgender women in the U.S. Women Health. 2014;54(8):750–67.
16. Knauer NJ. Same-sex domestic violence: claiming a domestic sphere while risking negative stereotypes. Temp Pol Civ Rts L Rev. 1998;8:325.
17. Stults CB, Javdani S, Kapadia F, Halkitis PN. Determinants of intimate partner violence among young men who have sex with men: the P18 Cohort Study. J Interpers Violence. 2019;
18. Messinger AM. Invisible victims: same-sex IPV in the national violence against women survey. J Interpers Violence. 2011;26(11):2228–43.
19. Flanders CE, Anderson RE, Tarasoff LA, Robinson M. Bisexual stigma, sexual violence, and sexual health among bisexual and other plurisexual women: a cross-sectional survey study. J Sex Research. 2019;12:1–3.
20. Copen CE, Chandra A, Febo-Vazquez I. Sexual behavior, sexual attraction, and sexual orientation among adults aged 18–44 in the United States: data from the 2011–2013 National Survey of Family Growth. Natl Health Stat Rep. 2016;88:1–4.
21. Anderson KL. Theorizing gender in intimate partner violence research. Sex Roles. 2005;52(11–12):853–65.
22. Wirtz AL, Poteat TC, Malik M, Glass N. Gender-based violence against transgender people in the United States: a call for research and programming. Trauma Violence Abuse. 2018;21(2):227–41.
23. Samons C. Same-sex domestic violence: the need for affirmative legal protections at all levels of government. S Cal Rev L So Just. 2012;22:417.

9 Intimate Partner Violence in the Military

Roger A. Mitchell

Case Review

Every day the medical examiner or forensic pathologist comes face to face with the end results of violence. Homicides and suicides are daily occurrences in cities and rural communities all over this country. This violence not only effects whole communities but finds much of its origins within families; between individuals. The forensic pathologist serves a vital role in providing the necessary context to the narrative surrounding violent death, particularly when it comes to domestic or intimate partner violence (IPV). Fatalities that result from IPV become the jurisdiction of the local medical examiner or coroner and are investigated to determine the cause and manner of death. The medical examiner for active service military personnel is the Armed Forces Medical Examiner located in Dover, Delaware. Deaths among veterans and their civilian spouses would be the jurisdiction of the local medical examiner or coroner. Over the last decade, in my forensic pathology practice, I have performed numerous death investigations and autopsy examinations on victims of IPV.

I will never forget the death case of a 32-year-old woman who was the girlfriend of an active duty military officer. The officer had just returned home from a tour of duty in the Middle East. According to neighbors and family members, he became overly possessive of his girlfriend with whom he lived. This was a new behavior for him that started upon his return. On several occasions, according to witnesses, he would show up at her job unannounced accusing her of being unfaithful. There were numerous 911 calls for domestic disturbances to the home over several weeks prior to the death. For example, on one particular evening, the neighbors heard loud arguing for several hours. The arguing was followed by high pitched screams from a woman. Upon arrival at the home, the death investigation revealed a young

R. A. Mitchell (✉)
Chief Medical Examiner of the District of Columbia, Washington, DC, USA
e-mail: roger.mitchel@dc.gov

R. K. Bailey (ed.), *Intimate Partner Violence*,
https://doi.org/10.1007/978-3-030-55864-2_9

African-American woman found face down in the vestibule of her home near her front door. She was wearing a blood soiled white and gray t-shirt with black leggings. She was bare foot with blood on the soles of her feet. There were two sets of bloody foot prints leading from the kitchen to the front door. One set of female bare foot prints and the other of boots, approximately size 11.

The autopsy revealed an African American woman in her late 20s to early 30s, approximately 5 feet 7 inches and 160 pounds with multiple stab wounds to the neck, chest, and back. There were approximately 20 stab wounds in total with several incised wounds to the hands and forearms indicating a defensive posture of the victim. There were several clusters of stab wounds to the left breast and right side of the back consistent with what is observed in intimate partner violence. The cause of death was determined as Multiple Sharp Force Injuries of the Neck and Torso.

The above case is a classic example of the type of homicide examined by the medical examiner in cases of domestic and intimate partner violence. It is also a good example of what may be seen in IPV among the military.

Introduction

The United States of America has a rich military history. From the American Revolution to the current conflicts in the Middle East, our soldiers have served our country with honor and distinction. This service has not come without significant sacrifice. Millions of families are separated for months and even years during war time. Fathers are separated from their children and wives are separated from their husbands. Service deployments have been documented to produce enormous amounts of stress for the military family that can often lead to divorce. Notwithstanding the effects on marriages, there are also a multitude of effects and consequences on the individual serviceman from the violence that accompanies war: consequences that ripple through all of our families, communities, and places of worship. According to the Defense Man Power Data Center (DMDC), in 2017, there were over 1.3 Million active-duty military in the United States Army, Navy, Marine Corps, Air Force, and Coast Guard [1]. The Veterans Administration reports that by September 2018, there will be over 19.2 million veterans living in the United States [2]. Our active duty and veteran men and women make up a large swath of our citizens, over 20 million, so it becomes extremely important that our public health, mental health, and healthcare delivery systems be properly equipped to serve this unique population.

Not so long ago in the summer of 2002, at Fort Bragg, North Carolina, the country was shocked by the murder of the wives of four Army soldiers. These women were killed shortly after their husbands returned home from war-time deployments. The intimate partner violence that proved fatal in these families occurred clustered within a 6-week period of each other. Three of the servicemen involved were members of the Special Operations units and had recently returned from Afghanistan. Two of those soldiers killed themselves. The fourth murder was by a sergeant from a regular Army unit that was not involved in the Afghan war. Several of these marriages were described as troubled and demonstrated the characteristics of ongoing and chronic domestic violence [3]. Three more women were murdered at Fort Bragg in 2008; this time they were female soldiers killed by a boyfriend or husband.

It is for these reasons why it is important to understand IPV in the military and how we can better serve our service men, women, and veterans. According to the Family Assistance Program (FAP) within the Department of Defense, an intimate partner has been defined as (1) a former spouse; (2) a person with whom the victim shares a child in common; or (3) a current or former intimate partner with whom the victim shares or has shared a common domicile. In such cases, the victim or the offender may have been an active duty service member or a civilian [4].

This chapter will focus on the distinctive expression of intimate partner violence among the military and their families. We will discuss the influence of adverse childhood experiences (ACE) and the link to post-traumatic stress disorder (PTSD) on the incidence and prevalence of IPV among this population. We will discuss the detection, treatment, and support opportunities for our military who are victims and even perpetuators of IPV. Lastly, we will discuss gaps and opportunities to improve the research and service delivery systems dedicate to decreasing intimate partner violence among the military.

Adverse Childhood Experiences

Adverse childhood experiences, also known as ACEs, can be defined as negative events, experiences, and/or incidents that occur during childhood that have the potential to adversely affect not only the child but also the adult that he or she will become. These include household dysfunction and neglect, as well as physical and emotional abuse. ACE can also include growing up in the home of a mentally ill or substance-abusing member of the household, witnessing domestic violence, experiencing parental divorce/separation, and/or having an incarcerated family member [5, 6]. What is most important is that the social environment in early childhood through adolescence has been proven to affect the physical and mental health outcomes in adulthood. It has been reported that childhood trauma has been associated with multiple psychiatric disorders in adults. ACE has been linked to depression, anxiety, substance abuse, and an increased risk of suicide attempts [5].

Imagine that you are a child who has experienced violence in your home, seen a family member murdered, or your father is incarcerated, and your mother has a substance abuse disorder. Imagine if you had an alcoholic father who abused you or sexually assaulted you. How would that effect your maturation? How would that effect your mental and physical health as an adult? What the adverse childhood experience research tells us is that a person who has experienced childhood trauma is at a higher risk of having cardiovascular disease at an earlier age with increased severity, and that person is at risk of obesity and diabetes in adulthood. What is most important, for the purpose of this chapter, is that the child is also at a higher risk of depression, anxiety, and suicide attempts in adulthood. It has also been suggested that childhood trauma also leads to a greater risk of post-traumatic stress disorder

(PTSD). We will come back to PTSD in the next section and its connection to IPV in the military. But for now, let's spend some time talking about ACE and the military. Some reports show that there is a higher percentage of people with childhood trauma who choose to join the military. One study found that servicemen reported higher exposure of nearly all forms of ACE when compared to the civilian responses and therefore suggested that military personnel have higher total burden of ACE [6]. Keep in mind that multiple ACEs have been reported to be cumulative on those who are affected. In other words, those who are exposed to numerous and different childhood traumas have higher risk of poor adult outcomes. Accordingly, those with one ACE have a 60–90% likelihood to suffer from additional ACE.

So why are soldiers more likely to have ACE exposures? It is possible that although many report that enlisting in the military service is for positive reasons such as patriotism and altruism, many soldiers may enlist in the military as an escape from childhood traumatic experiences and/or poor social environments. These men and women should be applauded for choosing military service as a way of changing their circumstances; however it is important to understand that this may prove to increase the burden of those suffering from childhood trauma who are enlisting in military service, therefore creating increased risk of developing physical and psychological illness among those affected servicemen and women. Because of the physical nature of becoming a soldier, there is less likelihood that the poor physical outcomes associated with ACE (i.e., hypertension, diabetes, obesity) will manifest themselves among these men and women [7]. The real risk to military personnel from the exposure to childhood trauma is the development of psychiatric illnesses such as stress, anxiety, depression, and post-traumatic stress disorder.

Post-Traumatic Stress Disorder

According to the National Institute of Mental Health (NIMH), post-traumatic stress disorder is defined as:

> A disorder that develops in some people who have experienced a shocking, scary, or dangerous event. It is natural to feel afraid during and after a traumatic situation. Fear triggers many split-second changes in the body to help defend against danger or to avoid it. This "fight-or-flight" response is a typical reaction meant to protect a person from harm. Nearly everyone will experience a range of reactions after trauma, yet most people recover from initial symptoms naturally. Those who continue to experience problems may be diagnosed with PTSD. People who have PTSD may feel stressed or frightened even when they are not in danger [8].

Diagnosis criteria of PTSD according to the DSM 5 include:

Criterion A: Stressor (One Required)

The person was exposed to death, threatened death, actual or threatened severe injury, or actual or threatened sexual violence, in the following way(s):

- Direct exposure
- Witnessing the trauma
- Learning that a relative or close friend was exposed to a trauma
- Indirect exposure to aversive details of the trauma, usually during professional duties (e.g., first responders, medics)

Criterion B: Intrusion Symptoms (One Required)

The traumatic event is persistently re-experienced in the following way(s):

- Unwanted upsetting memories
- Nightmares
- Flashbacks
- Emotional distress after exposure to traumatic reminders
- Physical reactivity after exposure to traumatic reminders

Criterion C: Avoidance (One Required)

Avoidance of trauma-related stimuli after the trauma, in the following way(s):

- Trauma-related thoughts or feelings
- Trauma-related external reminders

Criterion D: Negative Alterations in Cognitions and Mood (Two Required)

Negative thoughts or feelings that began or worsened after the trauma, in the following way(s):

- Inability to recall key features of the trauma
- Overly negative thoughts and assumptions about oneself or the world
- Exaggerated blame of self or others for causing the trauma
- Negative affect
- Decreased interest in activities
- Feeling isolated
- Difficulty experiencing positive affect

Criterion E: Alterations in Arousal and Reactivity

Trauma-related arousal and reactivity that began or worsened after the trauma, in the following way(s):

- Irritability or aggression
- Risky or destructive behavior
- Hypervigilance

- Heightened startle reaction
- Difficulty concentrating
- Difficulty sleeping

Criterion F: Duration (Required)

Symptoms last for more than 1 month.

Criterion G: Functional Significance (Required)

Symptoms create distress or functional impairment (e.g., social, occupational).

Criterion H: Exclusion (Required)

Symptoms are not due to medication, substance use, or other illnesses.

Two specifications:

- Dissociative Specification.
  - Depersonalization. Experience of being an outside observer of or detached from oneself (e.g., feeling as if "this is not happening to me" or one we are in a dream)
  - Derealization. Experience of unreality, distance, or distortion (e.g., "things are not real")
- Delayed Specification. Full diagnostic criteria are not met until at least 6 months after the trauma(s), although onset of symptoms may occur immediately [9].

The link between PTSD, the military, and exposure to combat related trauma is well established. Exposure to combat trauma has significant impact on service men and women. In research involving veterans deployed to Iraq and Afghanistan, investigators found that 44% of US soldiers suffered from PTSD, depression, or both after returning home from war [10]. There is a link between a soldier's exposure to childhood trauma in the form of ACE and the propensity of that soldier developing PTSD. Although, the literature does not suggest that childhood trauma and combat-related trauma are additive in their progression towards PTSD. It is being suggested that those soldiers with ACE exposure have a higher risk of developing PTSD after exposure to combat-related trauma, thus suggesting a cumulative relationship. Have you ever wondered why some veterans suffer from PTSD and others do not? It may be because those service men and women with PTSD may also have been exposed to trauma as a child or adolescent. Bremner et al. suggested that patients seeking treatment for combat-related PTSD have higher rates of childhood physical abuse when compared to combat veterans without PTSD [10]. The relationship between childhood trauma and combat-related trauma cannot be understated. Practitioners must understand this relationship in order to properly prevent and mitigate the development of PTSD and potentially intimate partner violence.

Intimate Partner Violence and the Military

Now that we have established that there is an interrelatedness between adverse childhood experiences, combat-related trauma, and PTSD, it is important to understand how these risk factors may influence the incidence of intimate partner violence among the military. In general, it has been reported that IPV among the military is greater than what is observed among the civilian population. Some reports suggest that IPV exists up to three times more than what is found in the civilian population. In a recent article published in Clinical Psychology Review, authors report the prevalence of IPV perpetuation among active duty servicemen and veterans range from 13.5% to 58%. This is a wide variation. Much of this variation can be suggested due to the wide variation of the presence of PTSD whether diagnosed or not [11]. The National Vietnam Veterans Readjustment Study (NVVRS) reported that an estimated 13.5% of veterans without PTSD perpetuated IPV during a given year compared to 33% of veterans with PTSD [12].

Although PTSD has been linked to intimate partner violence among service men, the occurrence of IPV within military families cannot be explained solely by a linear cause and effect paradigm described by the presence or absence of childhood trauma, combat trauma, and post-traumatic stress disorder. The family systems theory suggests that the occurrence of IPV in the military is complex and multifactorial with mutual influential causes [9]. Substance abuse, including alcohol use disorder, can play a part in intimate partner violence among the military. In one study 39% of veterans enrolled in an alcohol treatment program reported being perpetuators of IPV over a given year [2].

The number of deployments and frequency of deployments can also act as complex variables when attempting to understand the causative factors associated with IPV among this population. In one study it was reported that the longer the length of deployment, the greater likelihood of severe spousal violence in the military family. The deployment of the soldier is filled with many variables that can affect the family dynamic. The separation that accompanies deployment can produce anxiety and depression from the uncertainty of return and the uncertainty surrounding the strength of the relationship to withstand the separation. There is also a sense of loneliness that accompanies deployment, felt by both the spouse and the soldier. Much of these feelings are felt not only during the deployment but also during the pre-deployment phase [13]. When a soldier is preparing to leave his/her family, there is often emotional distance and withdrawal that occurs. Some families will tend to draw together pre-deployment. But still other families tend to draw apart. Both are intended to prepare the family for imminent separation. As a function of this separation, the family, including the soldier, will experience a series of emotions in the pre-deployment phase (i.e., stress, anxiety, depression). When the pre-deployment ritual is unhealthy, it can lead to increased anger, resentment, and arguing.

Much of the feelings that exist in the pre-deployment phase, both good and bad, may persist throughout the duration of the deployment and have the ability to affect the relationship satisfaction. In the cases where the soldier is leaving a family with young children, there is the potential for anger and resentment to be felt by the spouse. The single parenting that occurs during deployment therefore has the potential to influence relationship satisfaction. In a recent study conducted by Lara-Cinisomo et al., it was reported that caregivers who experienced more deployment separations reported lower relationship satisfaction, more hassles, and poor relationship well-being. Emotional stress felt during pre-deployment and deployment act as complex variables that have the potential to influence and act as risk factors for IPV in the military family [13].

But it is "coming home" that can be the most difficult for the military family. The post-deployment phase is filled with anxiety and emotional stress felt by the soldier and the spouse alike. The returning serviceman may or may not have encountered combat trauma while deployed. The trauma faced by the serviceman may be either physical or mental, both of which have their own set of issues. So, the emotional environment in the home, post-deployment, is important in understanding the potential risk of IPV. Data collected by Gibbs et al. and published in the 2012 edition of Military Medicine reveals that out of 20,166 records from married soldiers returning home from deployment, 3691 (18%) reported serious interpersonal issues [12]. In recent study performed, looking at general violent behavior among soldiers from the United Kingdom, 12.6% of the soldiers reported engaging in post-deployment violence [14]. If we are going to understand IPV between military families, it is important to look at the number of deployments, their duration, and their frequency. There is a real need within the military to ensure that there are adequate resources to support military families and their unique needs. If the United States military is going to be successful, then our soldiers and their families must be equipped with the mental and physical health to withstand the trials, barriers, and obstacles that comes with military service.

Family Advocacy Program

The Department of Defense – Office of the Secretary – is responsible for addressing domestic violence through the Family Advocacy Program (FAP). The FAP is mandated to respond to and prevent incidents of domestic violence for the military. The focus is on safety and risk management that includes (1) services to develop and monitor standardized risk management plans that ensure the safety needs of adult victims of domestic violence are met immediately; (2) establish standards for domestic abuse victim advocates who perform essential safety planning functions; and (3) establish standards for the involvement of military family advocacy services [14]. In addition, the program not only promotes prevention, early identification, reporting, and treatment of spouse abuse, but it is also established to preserve families in which abuse has occurred without compromising the health, welfare, and safety of the victims.

According to the DOD-FAP Report, there were 646,782 married couples in the military in FY2016. During that same fiscal year, there were 15,144 reported incidents of domestic/intimate partner violence. 8673 incidents met the criteria for domestic abuse or intimate partner violence. 73.8% were categorized as physical abuse, followed by 22.6% emotional abuse, 3.4% sexual, and nearly 1% neglect. Of the spouse abuse victims nearly half were military, the other half were non-military with 65% of the victims being female. 60% of the perpetuators were military. Just as important, 88% of the active duty offenders were male [4].

There are greater than 900 DOD-FAP licensed providers available to military families for treatment and case management. Reports are met with a 24/7 assessment and planning session that ensures the involvement of social services, medical treatment, and law enforcement. The IPV victim also receives clinical counseling and case management. The offender, too, receives an assessment as well as counseling and referral to case management. There is much emphasis placed on working with the offender within the FAP program – something that is not often witnessed within the civilian population. The equal emphasis on offenders may be due to the prevalence of the service man or woman as the perpetuator of the IPV. Clinical treatments for offenders include but are not limited to mental health services, substance abuse treatment, and anger management. Commanders can mandate treatment for active duty offenders, but the program is voluntary for active duty victims, civilian victims, and civilian offenders. For the program to be considered successful, FAP providers must show that there are no subsequent incidents that meet FAP criteria for greater than or equal to 75% of the participants. According to the recent FAP report, 95.9% of those receiving clinical services in FY2015 did not re-offend in FY2016 [4]. Could it be that the FAP program is that successful? That IPV in the military once recognized can be treated and the behavior corrected 95% of the time. It is not clear if the ongoing case management information reveals a 0% recidivism at year two, three, or even at year ten. There is more work to be done to ensure that offenders do not re-offend. The FAP also describes a comprehensive prevention program. FAP materials describe that there are pre-deployment support services for families as well as targeted efforts to address post-deployment stressors and family reunification. This includes education surrounding the adjustment and reunification stressors during post-deployment. Prevention efforts also include the training and educating of spouses on early warning signs of PTSD and traumatic brain injury (TBI). What is most important is that the larger military structure at the level of the Department of Defense has a recognized, funded, and operating support system for military families who are faced with intimate partner violence.

Case Example

Intimate partner violence among military families has forensic findings that are common. One common characteristic described in the case example in the beginning of the chapter is that many IPV cases include sharp force injury where the victim suffers "overkill." Multiple stab wounds to areas that are sexual in nature including the breasts or genitalia. The other common occurrence in the world of forensic pathology is the combination of homicide and suicide.

This next case is of a 25-year-old white man who was a soldier in a branch of the Armed Forces. He was recently married to his high school sweetheart. He has three children all under the age of 4 years old, one of which is a newborn. He had been deployed for 10 months this last time and was only home for 4 weeks between a previous 12-month deployment. He was allowed to come home and visit his newborn. His wife was a 23-year-old white woman who was a stay-at-home mother and the primary caregiver to her 1-month old son and 2-year-old and 3-year-old daughters.

The soldier was home for 2 weeks. There was no suggestion of any problems in the home. Law enforcement denies any history of calls for domestic disturbances. According to next of kin, he was known to be quiet and often would be uncomfortable in public settings. The mother of the spouse had not heard from her daughter in 2 days. That was unusual for her as she often required help with the children. The mother responded to the house only to find the 4-year-old crying in the kitchen on the floor, the 2-year-old in the playpen, and the 1-month old in the bassinet each crying out from hunger.

The scene was in a partially brick-front two-floor condominium with a drive-in garage. There was a set of steep steps up to the front door from the street. Entering the home revealed a well-kept home with a living room, kitchen, and family room. The children had already been removed by Youth and Family Services and were being placed with the grandmother.

The spouse was found in the master bedroom with a single gunshot wound to the right side of her head. She was clad in a night shirt and panties. There was blood soaked into the pillow and mattress under and near her head and upper torso. The soldier was found in the master bathroom just off the master bedroom with a single intra-oral gunshot wound. He is found sitting on the toilet slumped to the left with blood on the wall behind and above the toilet and a semi-automatic pistol on the tile floor near his right foot.

At the autopsy examination, the most important finding was the presence of stippling on the face and head of the woman indicating that the muzzle of the weapon was approximately 6 inches from her head when she was shot. The other important finding was the presence of soot on the upper hard palate in the mouth of the soldier indicating a close-range shot. The findings of both the soldier and his spouse are indicative of a murder-suicide. Homicide-suicide events are often seen among the military and law enforcement. These cases were certified as gunshot wound of the head and intra-oral gunshot wound of the head with manners of death suicide and homicide, respectively.

Conclusion

Cases of domestic and intimate partner violence are extremely sad. When it involves military families, who have sacrificed so much for this country, then this type of violence is even more disconcerting. We have learned so much about the risk factors that exist within intimate partner violence among the military. To understand why and how IPV occurs within military families, we must first understand what type of childhood the servicemen or women had. Were they exposed to violence as a child? Did they grow up in poverty? Did they have an incarcerated family member? Their childhood experiences can have either protective or risk properties to developing resiliency toward other future stress. And so, if we have new military recruits who have adverse childhood experiences, we must take the time to screen and assess their stress level. We must determine if they already have diagnosable depression and/or anxiety. At that point, upon their entry into the military, it is important to equip them with the tools to deal with their underlying mental health issues or stress. This must be done prior to exposure to combat-related trauma. This is particularly important in the pre-deployment phase. When the stress of the family is high due to the uncertainty that comes with the deployment to war or conflict, it becomes important for counselors and advocates working with the servicemen or women and their families underscoring the increased risk factors associated with combat deployment. Those servicemen or women with childhood trauma should be consistently reminded of their risk for a heightened response to combat-related stress. The family, particularly the spouse, should be involved with all the mental health support that occurs in enrollment into the military as well as any and all pre-deployment services.

Support services for the spouse and family that have been left behind are extremely important. As we now know, relationship satisfaction is an important protective factor to the development of IPV within a military family. Decreasing the stress of the caregiver allows for the servicemen or women to return to a low stress home environment post-deployment. There should be services in place to deal with the impact of multiple deployments on a family. The impact of multiple deployments as well as the length of deployments and their impact on the stress of the individual and family cannot be understated. Families must develop coping mechanisms to deal with consistent absence of the servicemen or women. Any support to assist in developing deployment resiliency is critical.

Deployed servicemen and women can be exposed to combat-related trauma. The trauma faced by the soldier can be either mental or physical. Preparing the soldier for what may be encountered is important in building individual resiliency. Mental health support should be made available to all that have been exposed to combat-related trauma, particularly those soldiers who have been identified to have suffered confounding childhood trauma. This type of support will lend itself to decrease incidence of PTSD. The spouse and family should also be equipped with the tools to recognize the signs and symptoms of PTSD post-deployment. Coming home can be difficult for the soldier, so helping the transition from war to home is important in mitigating the risk for intimate partner violence.

Investment in the mental health of servicemen and women is worth the cost. They have sacrificed so much for the liberty of our country. It is important for us to help protect military families from the IPV that tends to show its head in these stressful times. We owe them at least the service and support necessary to give them a chance at decreasing stress in them and in their homes. We can save a life and protect the future.

References

1. Defense Man Power Data Center (DMDC). DoD personnel, Workforce Reports & Publications. https://www.dmdc.osd.mil/appj/dwp/dwp_reports.jsp.
2. Williams JW. Department of veteran affairs: intimate partner violence: prevalence among U.S military veterans and active duty service-members and a review of intervention approaches; 2012.
3. Washington post https://www.washingtonpost.com/archive/politics/2002/07/27/slayings-of-4-soldiers-wives-stun-ft-bragg/0dbf9b27-6f99-4e91-9475-55255f4bd2c8/.
4. Family Advocacy Program (FAP) Report. Department of defense. Report on child abuse and neglect and domestic violence in the military for fiscal year 2016.
5. Hughes K, Bellis MA, Hardcastle KA, Sethi D, Butchart A, Mikton C, et al. The effect of multiple adverse childhood experiences on health: a systematic review and meta-analysis. Lancet Public Health. 2017;2(8):e356–66.
6. Katon JG, Lehavot K, Simpson TL, Williams EC, Barnett SB, Grossbard JR, et al. Adverse childhood experiences, military service, and adult health. Am J Prev Med. 2015;49(4):573–82.
7. Applewhite L, Arincorayan D, Adams B. Exploring prevalence of adverse childhood experiences in soldiers seeking behavioral health care during a combat deployment. Mil Med. 2016;181(10):1275–80.
8. NIMH. Post-traumatic stress disorder. https://www.nimh.nih.gov/health/topics/post-traumatic-stress-disorder-ptsd/index.shtml.
9. American Psychiatric Association. Diagnostic and statistical manual of mental disorders. 5th ed. Arlington, VA: American Psychiatric Association; 2013.
10. Bremner JD, Mishra S, Campanella C, Shah M, Kasher N, Evans A, et al. A pilot study of the effects of mindfulness-based stress reduction on post-traumatic stress disorder symptoms and brain response to traumatic reminders of combat in operation enduring freedom combat veterans with post-traumatic stress disorder. Front Psych. 2017;8(157)
11. Marshall AD, Panuzio J, Taft CT. Intimate partner violence among military veterans and active duty servicemen. Clin Psychol Rev. 2005;25(7):862–76.
12. Kulka R, Schlenger WE, Fairbank JA, Hough RL, Jordan BK, Marmar CR, Weiss DS. National Vietnam Veterans Readjustment Study (NVVRS). 1988. https://www.ptsd.va.gov/professional/articles/article-pdf/nvvrs_vol1.pdf.
13. Kelley ML, Stambaugh L, Milletich RJ, Veprinsky A, Snell AK. Number of deployments, relationship and perpetration of partner violence among U.S. navy members. J Fam Psychol. 2015;29(4):635–41.
14. Gibbs DA, Clinton-Sherrod AM, Johnson RE. Interpersonal conflict and referrals to counseling among married soldiers following return from deployment. Mil Med. 2012;177(10):1178–83.

Intimate Partner Violence Transcending Socioeconomic Class

10

Conte Terrell and Rahn Kennedy Bailey

In modern times, more women are in the workforce and contribute significantly to the household income. Does their financial independence have any influence on intimate partner violence (IPV)? In this chapter, we will explore if a woman's financial independence is protective. Indeed, it stands to reason, that one of the elements of coercive control employed by abusive partners (financial control), is eliminated. With separation, a victim of IPV who is financially independent would likely be able to support themselves and acquire housing, transportation, and other necessities. If a woman is more financially successful than her male partner, is he less likely to perpetrate abuse? Is the male partner cognizant of all her options and is she granted leverage over him? Perhaps a male partner may feel as though he doesn't have control or financial leverage and may resort to violence to gain "control" in a relationship.

Is there a relationship between IPV and money? Certainly financial dependence may restrict a victim's ability to leave an abusive relationship. Conversely, an abuser is often empowered by a victim's financial dependence. The autonomy of a victim is restricted when their abuser controls money within the relationship [1]. Financial instability has been thought to be the greatest reason why an abused woman returns to her abuser [1]. Thus, it becomes exceedingly important to understand that financial dependence is a tether that keeps a victim inexorably tied to their abuser. Law enforcement, family, and friends may indeed be successful in separating a victim from their abuser. However, if care is not taken to address the victim's needs of food, housing, healthcare, childcare, and transportation, an abuser may still maintain the

C. Terrell
Fresh Spirit Wellness for Women, Inc., Houston, TX, USA

R. K. Bailey (✉)
Department of Psychiatry, Charles R. Drew University of Medicine and Science, Los Angeles, CA, USA
e-mail: rahnkbaileymd@comcast.net

R. K. Bailey (ed.), *Intimate Partner Violence*,
https://doi.org/10.1007/978-3-030-55864-2_10

power to control and potentially abuse [1]. Sadly, this factor may lead a victim to accept reconciliation with her former abuser.

In 1900, the wage of a working married woman was less than that of a working child. And so it was young unmarried women and girls who were more likely to work during this time. Moreover, their earnings went to their parents [1].

However, black married women did work during this time (the 1900s). Their wages were low (equivalent to white children). This did not grant them financial equality in the home. Often there could be resentment from their husbands [1].

As women gained more education in the 1900s, they were directed into "feminine" jobs (nursing, librarian, and teacher). Even in the early 1900s, women had no claim to the wages they made. If married, her husband could claim her wages. In the 1940s college was becoming accessible – usually for middle-class and above women. Women's presence in the workforce was more prevalent after the 1950s with more women continuing to work after marriage. Only 18% of working women earned more than their working husbands in 1987 [1].

Socially, society's perspective is still "a woman should or will find a man to support her," and this may allow women to settle into situations where they are more likely to be financially dependent and so more easily coerced [1].

Additionally, many women today still are financially dependent on their partners [2]. Thus, financial inequity can shape roles in marriage or an intimate relationship. Even today childbearing and rearing may keep women away from the work force for prolonged periods. This can result in diminished economic power within a relationship. If there is inequity in pay or money that requires a woman to be financially dependent, this could place her at risk for maltreatment.

In the earliest times in the country, women were considered the property of their husbands. Thus, a woman's economic status was solely tied to the man she married. In colonial times, a woman's work was to be done within the context of the home. Society and her husband often imposed these norms. Though upward mobility was an option for husbands, it was not so for women. The case was far worse for African American women early in the country's history due to slavery. It was not until the mid-1800s that women were granted the right to own property. However, if she married, the control of the land reverted to her husband.

As mentioned earlier, financial dependence allows a victim to be controlled by a domineering partner.

Additionally, a financially, dependent victim may be likely to return to their partner if they are facing great economic hardship or homelessness without them. This may be complicated further with children. A woman may allow herself to be abused if this guarantees that her children are fed, clothed, and provided with shelter. Financial freedom, however, can provide protection from abuse. Evidence suggests abuse is reduced or prevented when a woman becomes less vulnerable and is active in the balancing of power within a relationship [3].

It seems that financial dependence is the main causative factor for women returning to their abuser [4]. It has been shown that male perpetrators of abuse exploit this to maintain control of their partner. Some abusers may cause their partner to be late for work. For example, they may show up at their partner's area of work and behave inappropriately in attempts to get them fired. This seems to be done in order to keep them financially dependent and isolated. An abusive partner may steal car keys to keep his victim in the house or allocate only meager amounts of money to her [4].

Throughout this book, it is noted that IPV is pervasive. All strata of society experience it. An important aspect of IPV perpetration is the abuser's ability to control and restrict resources both social and financial.

Indeed, sometimes, male partners may be resentful that their partner works. They usually seek to resolve this by limiting their partner's ability to work. This establishes the man as the primary earner and further isolates and controls the woman.

The race of the partners plays a role as well. White women are more likely than non-whites to be married. This makes them more closely linked to their abuser and harder to leave. The abuser can then find it is easier to limit their victims' work hours and/or access their accounts. The abusive husband may find it easier to conjure up reasons for his wife to stay at home and not work. I don't want my wife working/I need you home to take care of the kids. If a victim separates from her partner, she may face the daunting task of reentering the workforce. For highly skilled work, this could be problematic due to a prolonged absence from the workforce.

It seems that if a man can maintain coercive control over a woman and limit her access to funds, then income, education, or social status is not protective against IPV rates. However, if a woman is financially independent and is working, then she has greater ease and more options in regard to leaving. However, IPV is more complex than just finance. But it (financial independence) can aid when and if she decides to leave. Additionally, employment yields social support in the community and work force that may be helpful in reducing or escaping IPV [5].

The prevailing assumption is that economic empowerment is a potentially protective factor against IPV [6]. However, there are some theories that proclaim an associated risk of IPV even when a woman is a high earner. The relative resource theory [6] is a theoretical model that presumes that a man with limited resources (money, status, education) in a relationship will use violence as a resource to maintain control of a female partner. The theory has been interpreted to assume that a man who earns less than his female partner will feel as though his dominance and masculinity is threatened. However, many critics have pointed out that this theory neglects culture and gender views and generalizes men's behavior [7].

A competing view is that of marital dependence theory. This theory states that a woman who is financially dependent on their partner is more likely to be a victim of IPV. These two opposing theories were examined in a study in *The Journal of International* development titled How Does Economic Empowerment Affect Women's Risk of Intimate Partner Violence in Low and Middle-Income Countries? A Systematic Review of Published Evidence [7].

The study looked at indicators of women's economic empowerment. The indicators of empowerment included measures such as education and poverty. Looking at large cross-sectional studies, researchers sought to establish relationships with economic empowerment and IPV victimization among women. The study pointed out that higher socioeconomic status appeared to be protective against IPV victimization. However, the study reported an inherent bias – they asserted that stigma against IPV was higher among higher earners and may have led to underreporting [7].

Overall, this study bolsters the idea that access to education and the promotion of gender equality reduces the rate of IPV. This was found to be particularly true in the international community. The United Nations asserts that economic empowerment of women is protective against domestic violence [8].

Suffering abuse likely can keep a victim from work and reduce her earning power and independence [9]. Annually, the victims of domestic violence lost on average 7.2 days of work outside the home as a direct result of their injuries [10].

Does economic empowerment reduce the likelihood of women being victimized by their intimate partner? There are two opposing views on this matter. Some indeed believe that increased financial power protects women from abuse. Others, however, believe that with increased wages comes increased violence from intimate partners. Regarding the latter, it is believed to be a male compensatory mechanism enacted in response to a woman's associated status and independence [7]. In industrialized countries, the scientific consensus is that economic empowerment is protective against IPV [11].

In India, and perhaps other parts of the developing world, society has considered the man to be the sole economic provider. Moreover, women's work was considered to be mainly domestic and largely trivial. This may give males an undue sense of entitlement and superiority. This highlights the need for a change in the view of women and their role is society [12].

This social norm has seemed to carry over into people's collective thinking even if the woman works as well [12]. Importantly, the male partner's income relative to his female partner should be considered [12]. Sadly, in this particular study, wives who earn more than their husbands are more likely to be abused. Thus, IPV was provoked if a man's sense of superiority was challenged [13, 14]. It seems that in culture where antiquated views on women predominate, economic empowerment alone is not enough to protect against IPV. Economic empowerment needs to be coupled with increased social awareness to the harmful nature of domestic violence. Education is protective. Violence against an intimate partner (particularly a female) is unacceptable. This is a notion that society as a whole needs to adopt in order to enact true and lasting change/protection.

In conclusion, socioeconomic conditions seem to play a role as both a risk and protective factor regarding IPV. Trends show that if a woman achieves higher education, status, wages, and independence, she is less likely to be victimized in most circumstances. In areas of low education, mere financial empowerment is not protective. In fact, it may induce abuse from males who are resentful or fearful of a changing domestic dynamic. Like all things involving IPV, the situation is multifaceted. Domineering men can prevent their partner from accessing funds. This can create a situation effectively equivalent to financial dependence. There is the larger social and cultural ideology that may dictate an individual's role in a relationship. Society as a whole has been slow to grant women the same parity as men. However, vast increases in access to education have helped close this gap in many developed nations. Hopefully, increased education will help stymie abuse in developing countries as well. IPV is pervasive. Sadly, it is observed in all social strata. Women, in particular, have faced many hardships (both social and economic) that have encouraged their subjugation to men. Increased public awareness of IPV, along with efforts to promote gender equality, will hopefully reduce the incidence of partner violence in the future.

References

1. Conner DH. Financial freedom: women, money, and domestic abuse. Wm Mary J Women L. 2013;20:339.
2. Hornung CA, McCullough BC, Sugimoto T. Status relationships in marriage: risk factors in spouse abuse. J Marriage Fam, 1981;43(3):675–92.
3. Cunningham A, Jaffe PG, Baker L, Dick T, Malla S, Mazaheri N, Poisson S. Theory-derived explanations of male violence against female partners: literature update and related implications for treatment and evaluation. London: London Family Court Clinic; 1998.
4. Browne A, Salomon A, Bassuk SS. The impact of recent partner violence on poor women's capacity to maintain work. Violence Against Women. 1999;5(4):393–426.
5. Marmot M, Friel S, Bell R, Houweling TA, Taylor S. Closing the gap in a generation: health equity through action on the social determinants of health. Lancet. 2008;372:1661–9.
6. Choice P, Lamke LK. A conceptual approach to understanding abused women's stay/leave decisions. J Fam Issues. 1997;18(3):290–314.
7. Vyas S, Watts C. How does economic empowerment affect women's risk of intimate partner violence in low and middle income countries? A systematic review of published evidence. J Int Dev. 2009;21(5):577–602.
8. Dalal K. Does economic empowerment protect women from intimate partner violence? J Injury Violence Res. 2011;3(1):35.
9. Lyon E. Welfare, poverty, and abused women: new research and its implications. Harrisburg: National Resource Center on Domestic Violence; 2000.
10. Aizer A, Dal Bo P. Love, hate and murder: commitment devices in violent relationships. J Public Econom. 2009;93(3–4):412–28.
11. Macmillan R, Gartner R. When she brings home the bacon: labor-force participation and the risk of spousal violence against women. J Marriage Fam. 1999:947–58.
12. Krishnan S, Rocca CH, Hubbard AE, Subbiah K, Edmeades J, Padian NS. Do changes in spousal employment status lead to domestic violence? Insights from a prospective study in Bangalore, India. Soc Sci Med. 2010;70(1):136–43.
13. Rocca CH, Rathod S, Falle T, Pande RP, Krishnan S. Challenging assumptions about women's empowerment: social and economic resources and domestic violence among young married women in urban South India. Int J Epidemiol. 2008;38(2):577–85.
14. Schuler SR, Hashemi SM, Riley AP, Akhter S. Credit programs, patriarchy and men's violence against women in rural Bangladesh. Soc Sci Med. 1996;43(12):1729–42.

Gender Bias: The Male Victim

11

Terrence Schofield and Rahn Kennedy Bailey

In this chapter, the use of violence by women on their male partners will be examined. Women perpetrate the same level of physical and psychological abuse as men [1].

A substantial portion of individuals arrested for incidents of intimate partner violence (IPV) are women. Studies conducted across several states show that women comprise anywhere from 16–35% of those arrested [1]. Indeed, some of these women are ordered (via court-order) to attend services such as anger management. How do we know women commit violence at similar rates to men? This conclusion has been reached through the use of surveys. Interestingly, the National Family Violence Survey (1990) found that women reported higher rates of violence against their partners (relative to men) [1]. This may be in part due to fact that men are usually viewed as dishonorable if they admit perpetrating violence against a woman. Conversely, there is no such societal dictum in this regard toward women committing an act of violence on men. These factors likely influence how individuals self-report. When examining another type of violence, sexual coercion, women's behavior differs significantly from men. Sexual coercion is the use of threats (violent or psychological) to obtain sex that is not consensual. When examining this phenomenon, every study to date found that a higher percentage of men commit sexually coercive behaviors [1].

Indeed, one way that males and females differ in their perpetration of abuse regards the use of sexual coercion. Repeated throughout this book is the theme of a male perpetrator of abuse who uses verbal or physical threats to obtain sex from a non-consenting victim. This trend is not observed in women at rates that are

T. Schofield
Walden University, Minneapolis, MN, USA

R. K. Bailey (✉)
Department of Psychiatry, Charles R. Drew University of Medicine and Science,
Los Angeles, CA, USA
e-mail: rahnkbaileymd@comcast.net

R. K. Bailey (ed.), *Intimate Partner Violence*,
https://doi.org/10.1007/978-3-030-55864-2_11

comparable to men. In the National Violence Against Women Survey, both men and women reported being a victim of stalking [1]. However, women had a lifetime prevalence of 14.2% compared to 4.3% for men. Though women do stalk their intimate partners, the physiological burden of victimization tends to be more burdensome to female victims (according to self-reporting). Regarding stalking, women were 13 times more likely to report being "very afraid" of the stalker [1].

Psychological IPV is employed at equal rates between men and women. Acts of psychological aggression can be insulting, belittling, or demeaning comments that are indented to distress the victim [1]. However, the motive and context may be different.

That women perpetrate acts of violence at an equivalent rate may come as a surprise to many. Women do commit acts of violence and psychological abuse like their male counterparts [2]. However, unlike men, women tend to be less coercively controlling and perpetrate less acts of sexual aggression [3].

Coercion, the use of threats to isolate and control a victim is a behavior largely employed by men. This usually represents a desire to control the entirety of the relationship. Coercion, when used, is an implement of control and typical escalates in violence and severity. The violence that women perpetrate tends to stem more from a desire to influence a specific moment in a relationship. The violence is more sporadic and represents the desire to exact influence on a particular event (not the relationship and or partner as a whole). This type of non-coercive violence is seen perpetrated by men and women at equal rates. Despite the similar frequency and perpetration rates of violent aggression, women are reportedly injured far more often by acts of physical violence perpetrated by an intimate partner. This is thought to be owed to the size and strength disparity typically seen between men and women. In this book, there is an entire chapter devoted to examining IPV in the LGBTQ Community. See Chap. 8 for details on the complex dynamic of abuse among same-sex and its outcomes.

Not only are women who experience violence at a greater risk of physical injury, but the violence they perpetrate tends to be enacted as a response to violence perpetrated by their partner. Note that there are some states with mandatory arrest and/or persecution laws for domestic violence. This may put a battered woman in greater physical risk of injury and similar legal consequence risk as the primary perpetrator of abuse. A study found that acts of violence by women tended to be less severe even when compared to a retaliatory/reciprocal act of violence perpetrated by a man [4].

Women's use of violence in a relationship tends to be secondary to the violence she experiences at the hands of a male partner [5]. That is to say that the majority of women who perpetrate violence are victims of it as well. In relationships where both partners are violent, the term mutually violent has been used. In mutually violent relationships, women tend to experience more sexual abuse, coercion, domination, and injury [6]. Naturally, it is expected that women show greater psychological and physical ramifications from abuse [7].

The motivating factors for women committing violence against an intimate partner differ from men. Self-defense, fear, protecting children, and retribution are common motivations.

Most cases of violence against men in a heterosexual relationship occur in a mutually violent relationship. However, there is a group of men who are more vulnerable to one-sided abuse. Men with disabilities reportedly experience IPV at rates higher than men or women without disabilities [8]. Men with disabilities who experience abuse may feel stigma and not report abuse. They may fear the preserved indignity of being a man reporting abuse at the hands of a woman.

Additionally, if the intimate partner assists in the needs of daily living for the victim, then reporting abuse can present a real dilemma. Men with disabilities tend to visit doctors more frequently than men without disabilities, yet they may not report abuse due to the reasons given above. Similar to women suffering from abuse, men with disabilities have high rates of depression and stress-related symptoms that result from experiencing IPV [8]. An often forgotten-about portion of the male population reports a high incidence of IPV victimization. A study examining disabled men who received services from the Secret Garden, a disability-specific, nonresidential IPV program located in New York City, found that 66.2% of individuals in this group experienced abuse from an intimate partner. The majority of abuse reported in this particular study was physical violence. Due to their baseline health, many disabled men have frequent contact with healthcare professionals. Therein is a great opportunity for healthcare professionals to illicit information about disabled patients' health and safety. In fact, in 2012, 79% of adult men saw the doctor at least once. In that same year, nearly 90% of adult males visited the doctor at least once. Additionally, 29% of disabled men reported seeing the doctor more than 10 times per year [8].

Among men with disabilities, we see the intersection of two important issues regarding IPV and society. Men with disabilities may have little awareness of how to receive help. Perhaps they may be dependent on their partner for travel and so may be unable to seek aid inconspicuously. The second important burden men with disabilities face is the same burden that most abused men face. That is the burden of stigma and judgment. This is often coupled with the assumption that most people will not express sympathy or understanding regarding their plight [8].

It is important to note that unilateral violence against able-bodied men does occur as well. Cultural norms assert that a man's size and strength advantage over a woman deters violence. Furthermore, it is often believed that a man's relative size and strength is protective against violence perpetrated by a woman. However, this is not always true. Additionally, a woman may employ the use of weaponry to assault a male partner. Some men may feel it inappropriate to retaliate when a woman employs violence. A male may feel it is "unacceptable" to do so. "Real men should never hit a woman" is a phrase that is in society's collective conscious. Fear of violating these social norms may keep a man from retaliating or seeking outside help [9]. If a man responds to violence perpetrated by a woman with violence, he is often labeled as abusive. This label can be given even if the violent act was in self-defense.

Thus despite a size and strength advantage, a man may feel powerless in his relationship. Some abusive women have preemptively made threats to report their male partner to the police and make the claim that he is abusive if he makes any retaliatory action (even pushing to create distance) [9]. Some men believe that attempting to prevent their female partner's violence will incite more violence by her.

Rather than attempting to restrain or retaliate, some men may meet an act of violence with resignation in order to allow conflict to resolve. As referred to earlier in this chapter, violence perpetrated by women is often used to gain control or prompt a particular response from their partner in a particular moment or situation. Some men may view their partner's violent attack as the crescendo of psychological stress and tension. The inaction of violence then promises relief from the stress and tension of the current conflict.

There are some repeated themes expressed by men who are victims of IPV. Some themes echo the concerns abused women have, and some are more unique to men. Uniquely, some men express the need to maintain power (and control) in the relationship. This need to maintain control often serves as a deterrent to disclosing abuse. Some men feel as though disclosing abuse places/labels them as "a victim." For some men, victimization status identifies the abused man as one who has yielded power and control in the relationship. This can be seen as socially unacceptable and deter reporting. Indeed, some men may frame their abuse in ways they feel do not emasculate them.

Thus, masculinity, gender roles, and societal norms play significant roles regarding men and their decision on whether to seek help (and the way they express abuse) [9].

Often social stereotypes are woven into the personal stories of abused men. For example, many men deny having experienced pain during an assault. Even when men have filed orders of restraint against their abuser, it is often framed as a power-play or cunning tactical decision. Indeed, more assertive and masculine attributes are credited to their decision-making, and fear is often not mentioned or is minimized. Some men have even described having experienced objective sexual coercion against them.

However, most men are reluctant to frame it as such. These types of outward displays of bravado make it difficult to gauge the full spectrum of abuse men experience and its ill effects [10]. This is important because it informs how society (law, studies, etc.) views the issue of male victims of IPV. This may have an influence on the figures of men (self-reporting) sustaining trivial injuries and low psychological impact when compared to women victims of abuse.

There has been some progress regarding honest disclosure of abuse and the associated ill effects. In some studies, men were allowed to share their experience in a way that allowed them to define IPV and abuse.

The men in this study expressed the typically diametrically opposed views of experiencing fear while denying victimization and loss of control [10]. The fear of injury was reported. Men have said that women's ability to inflict physical injury is comparable to that of a man.

However, the problem is usually compounded because often men are afraid to defend from the attack. Some men even expressed fear that their partner may kill them while still feeling unable to defend themselves.

The allowance for the appearance of maintaining power and control in a relationship can give an abused man his own framework in which to disclose abuse. Under these conditions, men often give stories anathema to the typical "men do not fear intimate partners" reports stated earlier in this chapter. Sensitivity to victimization and its stigma play important roles in how a man is likely to report abuse. This should be taken into consideration when eliciting information from a man who is likely being abused.

Norms of masculinity can color abuse. It can be a source of pride that despite being physically attacked, a man has never hit his partner. A man may frame it in a way that attempts to portray him as in control. Sentiments like "I could have hit her, but did not" highlight a man's control and benevolence and downplay victimization. Therefore, they tend to appear more in the narrative of the abused man. He is not a victim; he is a stoic and chivalrous man who is protecting his woman by not harming her during her insignificant tantrums.

There is a belief among most men that certain characteristics are inherently masculine. These characteristics are dominance, power, control, and strength. These characteristics extend into the domain of relationships where it is believed a man should be dominant and in control. Research supports allowing men to express their abuse in a way that conforms to their individual identity of masculinity.

Calling the authorities is often seen as a "lose-lose" proposition by many men. An average of 1.6 million domestic violence incidence occurred between 2006 and 2015. The police were involved in approximately 56%. During these interactions with authorities, an arrest or criminal charges resulted in 39% of the cases [11]. As stated earlier, men tend not to seek the aid of the police for two major reasons. Either the act of seeking help/calling the police is viewed as unmanly and is in itself unacceptable, or the victim believes he will be viewed as/labeled as the batterer [12, 13]. Many male victims may have felt assault should go unreported stating the matter was "minor or unimportant [14]. However, women can initiate violence [15]. More support and infrastructure is needed for male victims [16].

Lastly, there are incidences of women killing their male intimate partner. Usually such homicide occurs in the backdrop of domestic disharmony [17]. A study examining homicides perpetrated by wives highlights that in those relationships that ended in homicide, there was a long history of violence and abuse. Weather the relationship was mutually abusive was not elucidated. However, police reports show that 71% of the cases examined were victim-perpetrated. That is to say, the wife felt threatened or was initially attracted by the husband. Thus we do see in this example incidences of wives killing their husbands. However, the female does not seem to be the initiator in the actions that ultimately lead to homicide.

In fact, research supports the notion that women are more psychologically aggressive than men in relation to male IPV. Research stated two studies that examined the psychological aggression and physical violence of women, concluded that "women use higher levels of moderate physical violence than their partners used against them and about the same level of severe physical violence," [18]. Male victims of IPV may experience broken limbs, stab wounds, teeth marks, deep scratches and lacerations, inappropriate comments, fear and intimidation, and emotional aggression. Consequently, these male victims may refuse physical examination by nurses, particularly female nurses, or seek the support of health professionals and services [19].

Some continue to see IPV as a predominantly female issue, but research has proven that within the United States IPV is pervasive, with an estimated 4.7 million women and 5.4 million men victimized yearly at a cost to health systems of $2.3 billion to $7.0 billion [20]. We particularly will look at concepts of self-identity, masculinity and gender roles, in relation to IPV as contributors to IPV among African American males.

Self-Identity

In terms of identity formation, how one perceives themselves and their reactions to others is a major contributor in their personal self-identity formation. The self is a term used to describe how a person acts socially in their own company and in the presence of others, a view of self as a process [21]. Furthermore, individuals can view themselves in many ways, and this view of self is developed through social interactions and gradually determines how the individual interacts with others [22].

How males self-identify power and masculinity is a major contributor to how they perceive violence in intimate relationships. Male control over women is one way men demonstrate and enforce their masculine identity [23].

The provider image in how men self-identify challenges the root of their masculinity and identity. Unresolved feelings are a major contributor to unsettled anger and violent behaviors. For example, men may struggle to attain a masculine ideal of "provider" when jobs are scarce, leaving few options for demonstrating masculinity other than through violence against other males and female partners [24].

The way we are reared contributes to the way we justify and exhibit violent aggression. Growing up in an abusive household may normalize violence, resulting in reinforcement of harmful masculinity norms and intergenerational replication of IPV [25].

Furthermore, how a male develops violence has a strong correlation to their social adaptation to major events in life. Those with low self-esteem are vulnerable to high levels of rejection sensitivity or to basing self-worth on others' acceptance of them. They may anxiously expect, perceive, and overreact to rejection, and react unfavorably to avoid it. In relationships, men may react with hostility, jealousy, or attempts to control partners, while women can withdraw from supports and become despondent when faced with the possibility of rejection [26].

Males are particularly self-identified and strongly associated with masculine power and control. Research suggests that power and control are often defined for men within the context of the construction of masculinity. For example, "being a real man" may include the ability to assert power and control over others and a man's perceived value may be tied to the amount of power and control he has over others. When a man internalizes this notion of masculinity and links his own value to the amount of power and control he has, he may use violence against his partner. He does this to regain back the power he perceives as being threatened [27].

Our judicial system feeds false perceptions of male IPV victimization and a major contributor to how males self-identify as the perpetuator of IPV violence. A court report study found that almost one-half (47%) of the cases involving women arrested for domestic violence against a male intimate partner were rejected by prosecutors, and another 16% had been dismissed by a judge. Legal factors, such as a defendant's prior criminal arrests, use of a weapon, victim injury, and, most important, the type of arrest (dual vs. single arrest), all affected prosecutors' decisions in these cases. Female defendants arrested for offending against a male intimate partner were treated more leniently than male defendants or women arrested for domestic offenses involving other types of relationships [28].

Masculinity

Our gender roles have a lot to do with how we exhibit violence among our partners. Research suggests socially constructed norms and beliefs surrounding masculinity, femininity, and how women and men interact in sexual relationships are important constructs for understanding the etiology of young men's use of violence against a female partner. Among African American men, masculinity is culturally designed to define what it means to be masculine and manliness. In addition, studies show that young Black men may integrate culturally specific notions of manhood into their conceptions of masculinity, "drawing on fragments of the dominant masculinity [and] piecing together aspects of it to establish their own standards and meanings" [29].

One of the major masculine issues of IPV among males is maintaining a sense of honor in justifying IPV acts. Honor norms require men to be hypersensitive to insults and threats to their reputation, and a key component of the masculine reputation is the good name of a man's female partner. Thus, honor culture softens established norms where female chastity, purity, and modesty are valued, as emphasized in an Arab expression that a man's honor "lies between the legs of a woman" [30].

Because male honor often requires female deference and fidelity, relationships between men and women can carry an underlying tension that can serve as a precursor or catalyst to domestic violence. Honor may be used as a justification (either implicit or explicit) for violence; in the most extreme cases, it is used as a justification for homicides of spouses or family members in honor cultures [31].

Male viewpoints of masculinity contribute to their ideology of violence. Socially constructed ideologies about masculinity from the things they encounter from institutional racism, and the expectations and beliefs about what men should do, or what attributes they should perform, are implicated in men's perpetration of violence. Research suggests that anger, hatred, and frustrations of African American men from institutional racism are projected onto African American women [32].

Research on identity and behavioral expression stated that men who internalize ideals of manhood as defined by aggression, dominance, and toughness are more likely to abuse female partners [33].

Masculinity and victimology are strange bedfellows and create dysfunctional adjustment and attachment responses within toxic IPV relationships. Research suggests that the traditional ideal of "manliness" still influences attitudes and beliefs from others. Additionally, those who have been sexually abused themselves judge themselves by this ideal which doesn't allow for a male to be a victim [34].

Additionally, there are some men who also appear to choose more stereotypically masculine reasons for remaining in intimately violent relationships (e.g., being seen as a failure and children needing both parents), yet both males and females were more likely to internally justify to themselves rather than externally to others [35].

Masculine discrepancy stress and failure to conform to socially male-conformed norms can tint aggressive behaviors and present future IPV rooted behaviors. Research suggests that the possibility of negative effects of harmful masculinity occurs when negative masculine ideals are upheld and masculine discrepancy stress from failure of fulfilling male-conformed norms predict the perpetuation of men's IPV behavior [36].

Gender Roles

Research suggests that among African American males, "gender roles influence the way [young Black] men understand and engage educational opportunity, labor force participation, and relationships with women and other men…limiting conceptions of opportunity and success and exposing some to stigmatization, abuse and violence" [37].

Measures of gender views encompassed multiple sub-domains of specific content areas, such as male beliefs of sexual entitlement, control over wealth, and the acceptability of use of violence against women, either as a demonstration of masculinity or to enforce traditionally defined gender roles for girls and women [38].

Our societal norms deny IPV experiences of male IPV survivors. The reaction of the community members and service providers to male survivors of sexual assault was very much dependent on the survivor's sexual orientation and the gender of the perpetrator. This suggests that societies view on who can be a victim is still influenced by how an individual identifies themselves sexually, an unsettling thought in present times [39]. These gender perspectives and societal norms challenge the realization if male IPV victimization truly exists. If men are not typically considered within the dominant discourse on IPV, experiences of IPV stigmatization may be compounded with the perception that men are not victims of IPV. Thus minority men experience more perceived stress due to exposure to racial and other stressors, and thus, IPV may be stronger among ethnic minority men [40].

If gender norms are the measuring rod, then what it means to be a man has already been defined by who I see to what men become. Thus, men may have similar concerns about anticipated and internalized stigma but may face additional barriers, such as legitimizing their experiences of partner abuse [41].

Most males see themselves as masculine and females subordinate to the masculine, which will prompt gender male superiority as a form of justifying violent responses. Research suggests being defied or shown up by an "insubordinate" female partner, or otherwise having her publicly challenge his authority—can be seen as the height of unmanliness and justification for a violent response [42].

Male gender role conflict is the motivator behind behavioral and personality expressions. Research supports this view stating that gender-role conflict may result in the "need" for the individual experiencing the conflict to assert his membership in that gender group by displaying exaggerated examples of gender-appropriate behavior. The ways in which masculinity is typically understood may predispose men to IPV against women. Some of the traditional aspects of the construction of masculinity include masculinity status which is how a man must gain respect of others, toughness, male expectation that all men are supposed to be physically tough and aggressive, and lastly, anti-feminine, meaning a masculine man does not engage in acting feminine or participate in any type of stereotypical feminine roles [43].

The socialization of masculine ideals starts at a young age and defines ideal masculinity as related to toughness, stoicism, heterosexism, self-sufficient attitudes, and lack of emotional sensitivity [44].

In closing, it is important to understand that in heterosexual relationships, IPV against men does occur. There are strong cultural attitudes that define what a man should be. Many abused men do not want to violate this norm. They may go to great lengths to frame their relationship (however abusive) as one in which they maintain power and control. Society's expectations of men have influenced how they discuss abuse and ironically perpetuate the often false narrative of the stoic man in the public zeitgeist. Allowing men to share their experience without labels such as "victim" yields the greatest insight into his relationship.

He may not identify with the term victim because he truly feels he is not one. He may view himself as a courageous man with an iron constitution who is resolute in his commitment to never strike a woman. Therefore, some tailoring of questioning and awareness to social mores needs to be taken into account while having discourse with a male victim of abuse. They may view their suffering as noble, and they may feel as though inaction is the most honorable option. More is needed to understand the abused men's perspective. Allowing him to voice his experience in a way that lets him preserve his masculine identity seems to be a good approach.

References

1. Swan SC, Gambone LJ, Caldwell JE, Sullivan TP, Snow DL. A review of research on women's use of violence with male intimate partners. Violence Vict. 2008;23(3):301–14.
2. Straus MA. The controversy over domestic violence by women: a methodological, theoretical, and sociology of science analysis. In: Arriaga XB, Oskamp S, editors. Violence in intimate relationships. Thousand Oaks: Sage; 1999. p. 17–44.

3. Johnson MP. Conflict and control: gender symmetry and asymmetry in domestic violence. Violence Against Women. 200;12(11):1003–18. https://doi.org/10.1177/1077801206293328.
4. Belknap J, Melton H. Are heterosexual men also victims of intimate partner abuse. Harrisburg, PA: VAWnet, a project of the National Resource Center on Domestic Violence/Pennsylvania Coalition Against Domestic Violence, 2005.
5. Johnson MP. Patriarchal terrorism and common couple violence: two forms of violence against women. J Marriage Fam. 1995;57:283–94.
6. Dasgupta SD. A framework for understanding Women's use of nonlethal violence in intimate heterosexual relationships. Violence Against Women. 2002;8(11):1364–89. https://doi.org/10.1177/107780102237408.
7. Afifi TO, MacMillan H, Cox BJ, Asmundson GJG, Stein MB, Sareen J. Mental health correlates of intimate partner violence in marital relationships in a nationally representative sample of males and females. J Interpers Violence. 2009;24(8):1398–417. https://doi.org/10.1177/0886260508322192.
8. Ballan MS, Freyer MB, Powledge L. Intimate partner violence among men with disabilities: the role of health care providers. Am J Mens Health. 2015;11(5):1436–43.
9. Allen-Collinson J. A marked man: female-perpetrated intimate partner abuse. Int J Mens Health. 2009;8(1):22–40. https://doi.org/10.3149/jmh.0801.22.
10. Brooks C, Martin S, Broda L, Poudrier J. "How many silences are there?" Men's experience of victimization in intimate partner relationships. J Interpers Violence. 2017:886260517719905. https://doi.org/10.1177/0886260517719905. [Epub ahead of print]
11. Reaves BA. Police response to domestic violence, 2006–2015. Washington, DC: Bureau of Justice Statistics; 2017.
12. Mille SL, Meloy ML. Women's use of force: voices of women arrested for domestic violence. Violence Against Women. 2006;12(1):89–115. https://doi.org/10.1177/1077801205277356.
13. Corbally MA. Making sense of the unbelievable: a biographic narrative study of men's stories of female abuse (Master's thesis). England: University of Salford; 2011.
14. Corbally M. Accounting for intimate partner violence: a biographical analysis of narrative strategies used by men experiencing IPV from their female partners. J Interpers Violence. 2015;30(17):3112–32. https://doi.org/10.1177/0886260514554429.
15. Hines DA, Brown J, Dunning E. Characteristics of callers to the domestic abuse helpline for men [electronic version]. J Family Violence. 2007;22:63–72.
16. Dobash RP, Dobash RE. Women's violence to men in intimate relationships. Br J Criminol. 20044;44:324–49.
17. Goetting A. Homicidal wives: a profile. J Family Issues. 1987;8(3):332–41. https://doi.org/10.1177/019251387008003006.
18. Barber C. Domestic violence against men. Nursing Standard. 2008;22(51):35–9.
19. Henning K, Renauer B. Prosecution of women arrested for intimate partner abuse. Violence Vict. 2005;20:171–89.
20. Black M, Basile K, Breiding M, Smith S, Walters M, Merrick M, et al. The National Intimate Partner and sexual violence survey (NISVS): 2010 summary report. Atlanta, GA: National Center for Injury Prevention and Control, Centers for Disease Control and Prevention; 2011.
21. Blumer H. Symbolic interactionism: perspective and method. New Jersey: Prentice Hall; 1969.
22. Carter M, Fuller C. Symbols, meaning, and action: the past, present, and future of symbolic interactionism. Curr Sociol. 201;64(6):931–61.https://doi.org/10.1177/0011392116638396
23. Fleming PJ, McCleary-Sills J, Morton M, Levtov R, Heilman B, Barker G. Risk factors for men's lifetime perpetration of physical violence against intimate partners: results from the international men and gender equality survey (IMAGES) in eight countries. PLoS One. 2015;10:e0118639. PMID:25734544
24. Jewkes R, Morrell R. Gender and sexuality: emerging perspectives from the heterosexual epidemic in South Africa and implications for HIV risk and prevention. J Int AIDS Soc. 2010;13:6–6. PMID:20181124
25. Heise LL. Violence against women: an integrated, ecological framework. Violence Against Women. 1998;4:262–90.

26. Crocker J, Park L. The costly pursuit of self-esteem. Psychol Bull. 2004;130:392–414.
27. Harway H, O'Neil JM. What causes men's violence against women? Thousand Oaks: Sage; 1999.
28. Willie T, Kershaw TS. Associations between latent classes of interpersonal poly victimization and Polyperpetration and sexual risk behaviors among young pregnant couples: a dyadic analysis. Arch Sex Behav. 2018;47(6):1699–709. https://doi.org/10.1007/s10508-018-1183-x.
29. Ruxton S. Man-made: men, masculinities and equality in public policy. London: Coalition on Men and Boys. https://www.menshealthforum.org.uk/man-made-men-masculinities-and-equality-public-policy. 2009.
30. Beyer L. The price of honor. Time, 55, January 18, 1999.
31. Abou-Zeid A. Honour and shame among the Bedouins of Egypt. In: Peristiany J, editor. Honour and shame: the values of Mediterranean society. London: Weidenfeld & Nicholson; 1965. p. 243–59.
32. Hampton RL, William O, Magarian L. Domestic violence in the African American community: an analysis of social and structural factors. Violence Against Women. 2003;9:533–57.
33. Anderson E. Code of the street: decency, violence, and the moral life of the Inner City. New York: W. W. Norton & Company; 1999.
34. Andersen TH. Against the wind: male victimization and the ideal of manliness. J Social Work. 2011;13(3):231–47.
35. Eckstein JJ. Reasons for staying in intimately violent relationships: comparisons of men and women and messages communicated to self and others. J Family Viol. 2011;26(1):21–30.
36. Reidy DE, Berke DS, Gentile B, Zeichner A. Man enough? Masculine discrepancy stress and intimate partner violence. Personal Individ Diff. 2014;68:160–4. https://doi.org/10.1016/j.paid.2014.04.021.
37. Littles MJ, Bowers R, Gilmer M. Why we can't wait: a case for philanthropic action: opportunities for improving life outcomes for African American males. New York: Ford Foundation; 2007.
38. Raiford JL, Seth P, Braxton ND, DiClemente RJ. Interpersonal- and community-level predictors of intimate partner violence perpetration among African American men. J Urban Heal. 2013;90:784–95.
39. Davies M. Male sexual assault victims: a selective review of the literature and implications for support services. Aggress Viol Behav. 2002;7(3):203–14.
40. Gordon DM, Moore KE, Vincent W, Iwamoto DK, Campbell C, Hunter BA, et al. Intimate partner violence among low-income fathers: testing a stress-coping model. J Interpers Violence. 2017:886260517736878. https://doi.org/10.1177/0886260517736878. [Epub ahead of print]
41. Overstreet N, Quinn D. The intimate partner violence stigmatization model and barriers to help seeking. Basic Appl Soc Psych. 2013;35(1):109–22.
42. Miller J. Getting played: African American girls, urban inequality, and gendered violence. New York: NYU Press; 2008.
43. Vincent W, Gordon DM, Campbell C, Ward NL, Albritton T, Kershaw T. Adherence to traditionally masculine norms and condom-related beliefs: emphasis on African American and Hispanic men. Psychol Men Masc. 2016;17(1):42–53. https://doi.org/10.1037/a0039455.
44. Wall D, Kristjanson L. Men, culture, and hegemonic masculinity: understanding the experience of prostate cancer. Nurs Inq. 2005;12:97.

12 Intimate Partner Violence in Male-Dominant Sports Culture

Derek H. Suite

Case Illustration

John is a star player on his current team. As a model player, John is always on time, or early, for practice and enjoys a reputation of working harder than any of his teammates on the field. He has a supportive, sports-centered family. His dad played football, his brother played basketball, and his mom coaches high school basketball. John is engaged to his "best friend," Marcia. She recently relocated to live with John, at his request, because he wanted her support as he was away from home.

In his third season seemingly at the height of his success, John sustained a season-ending injury that required multiple surgeries and approximately 6 months of physical therapy before he could be deemed fit to resume playing. During this period his teammates and team staff noticed that John appeared distracted and was no longer energetic and upbeat. From usually energetic and gregarious, John became isolative and minimally communicative—giving mostly one word answers when coaches and trainers approached him. John was referred to a sports psychologist to help support him as he coped with his disabling injury. In session, John admitted to feelings of inadequacy and guilt that he let his team down by getting injured. He was quite frustrated with the team losing games while he was injured and also blamed himself for the losses. He stated he was worried that he may not play again for the rest of the season and wondered if this would affect his contract going forward. He admits that he feels powerless and useless and that these are strange feelings for him.

When asked about how he copes with his anxieties and frustrations, John stated that he likes to exercise but could not do so because of the injury, so he stays up late most nights playing video games and sometimes smokes "weed," approximately 2 to

D. H. Suite (✉)
Teachers College, Columbia University, New York, NY, USA
e-mail: drsuite@fullcirclehealthny.com

R. K. Bailey (ed.), *Intimate Partner Violence*,
https://doi.org/10.1007/978-3-030-55864-2_12

3 times a week. John endorsed smoking weed to calm down, especially if "I'm super stressed," "in pain," or "when my girl is getting on my nerves."

John endorsed occasionally drinking alcohol, mostly with his teammates once or twice a week, but admits later on that he has had a few drinks on occasion by himself when he is feeling down and especially when he feels the recovery process is going too slow. When queried about triggers for his stress other than not playing, John initially says, "nothing really." He is reminded that he mentioned using weed and alcohol to calm down when his fiancé got on his nerves. John responds, "Oh yes, but it's no big deal. We have known each other for years and know how to push each other's buttons. It gets real nasty sometimes but we always make up."

When asked how nasty things get between him and Marcia, John stated, "really bad when I am drunk but after a couple of days we always make up." With further prompting, John admitted that he has pushed Marcia a few times—and a couple of times prevented her from leaving the bedroom forcibly holding her in place. He added that the violence was not one-sided. He emphasized, "Doc, I am telling you she is really aggressive with the mouth." When asked why he resorted to physical violence, John stated, "that's the only thing she understands; she knows how I get and she pushes me. It's like she wants it." John recalled some of his teammates telling him to "be careful" about hitting Marcia after they witnessed him "smacking her around a couple of times when I was real drunk" but stated "I never got around to it because things always get better." John admitted that he sometimes "felt really bad" and "guilty" about being violent with Marcia because "she is such a nice girl. She would do anything for me." He also added that he was advised by some vets on the team that his behaviors will change once he starts playing again.

When asked about what he thinks might be at the root of his violent behaviors, John initially could not think of any possible triggers, other than stating "I guess I am just that kind of guy." He did endorse seeing his father and older brothers engage in violent behaviors against women and added that he thought that in some cases, "they really deserved it" because they were "too aggressive." He gave several examples of women in his family "provoking" fights by saying derogatory remarks to their husbands. He added that many of the women in his family "hit first." He recounted a story of his youngest sister hitting him and his having to forcibly grab her and pin her down while shaking her and reminding her "I am a man, what are you doing; you gonna make me snap."

When asked about what might be going on currently that contributes his potential to become violent, John cited the frustrations of having to be home more (which he was not used to) because of the injury, the negative effect of the team losing games, and Marcia's lack of understanding of his level of stress combined with her constant nagging and bossy attitude. In John's mind, these stressors created a "perfect storm" that pushed him to become violent toward her. Marcia's attempts to retaliate by hitting him back further escalated the problem, per John's report, because "it made me lose control more. I can't let any woman hit me, especially in front of other people." John is asked about his interests in obtaining help for his violent behaviors. He inquired if he and Marcia can come in for couples counseling and was informed that it would be best if Marcia could come in for a session on her own. John agreed to this and to coming in for individual counseling to address his negative coping and substance use. He was encouraged to take a referral to attend an IPV program. He expressed a strong reluctance to attend an IPV group program for fear of being recognized. John stated that he does not want to lose his job if the team or the league finds out. He did not want to disappoint his fans: "millions of people--especially kids—look up to me; I can't let them down." The consequences and negative outcomes of not getting immediate help were discussed with John.

Marcia was seen individually and admitted to being physically assaulted repeatedly by John but stated she was "in love" with him and not ready to leave him. She divulged that she was 1 month pregnant and waiting on the right time to tell John. Marcia stated she believed that John will change once she told him the "good news" that she was "carrying his child and he would soon be a father." Marcia is counselled on the realties associated with untreated IPV and its effects on pregnancy and children. She accepted a referral for an individual counselor and signed a release so that the counselor can be informed of the findings of her initial session.

Despite agreeing to see a counselor, Marcia eventually decided she no longer wanted to follow up with a counselor. When queried about her reasoning, she stated she did not think "this was a big deal" and did not want matters to get "out of hand" and jeopardize John's career and their future. When asked about her safety, Marcia responded that, despite the violence, she "never felt unsafe" and indicated she knows how to fend for herself because she has had to deal with, what she termed, "men being men" all her life. She shared that she grew up watching her father become physically and verbally abusive to her mother and stated they "never separated or divorced", but worked through the trouble with the help and support of their church. She added that she liked the life that she and John had built and that he takes good care of her (he does not want her to work). She stated that there was nothing John wouldn't give her—but she would never ask for much anyway.

John did eventually attend an individual session with his team's mental performance clinician and agreed to a treatment and accountability plan to attend individual sessions with an external counselor to work on his accountability issues. Because he did not want his team to be made aware, John repeatedly refused offers to voluntarily enroll in a formal DV program. He did not want his insurance provider to be alerted that he was in an anti-violence program and decided to self-pay external counseling sessions with a provider who had experience with DV.

Within the first 3 weeks of therapy, John complained that the external counselor, though "a nice guy," did not understand the dynamics and pressures associated with his being a professional athlete. Nevertheless, John reported making significant progress at home with no incidences of violence but a month later found himself the subject of several news articles detailing that his wife had filed a police report and took out an Order of Protection against him.

Although Marcia later recanted and dropped charges against John, stating that she "made the whole thing up," his team suspended him, and he became the subject of a league investigation. Several months later, it was determined that John, in light of the charges being dropped; his wife's recanting of her allegations; and his willingness to obtain help, would be suspended for five games the following season with the stipulation that he remain engaged in 6 months of professional domestic violence counseling. When subsequently interviewed by the media, John stated that he was focused on "getting himself better, taking care of his family, and helping the team."

John's situation, subsequent to the suspension, became more complicated after the media published a story that two women from his past alleged previous violent experiences with him.

Overview

John and Marcia's case illustration, with its vexing cycle of love, power, control, fear, intimidation, violence, guilt, forgiveness, and hope, is not unique to sports culture. Many couples, within the United States, and indeed around the world, struggle to cope with the vexing cycle of intimate partner violence (IPV). Although IPV has already been defined elsewhere in this book, it is worth emphasizing that IPV is a significant "public health issue" with serious, negative physical and psychological health outcomes [1, 2, 3, 4, 5].

IPV poses significant social and public health costs [6, 7, 8]. It is within the larger context of IPV as a widespread, public health phenomenon that insights and observations about its manifestation within sports culture are explored within this chapter.

At the outset, it is duly noted that the underlying psychosocial factors and sociocultural forces that contribute to the incidence of IPV are pervasive within society. Little to no available research studies conclusively demonstrate that athletes who commit IPV did so as a result of being involved in their sport. Despite the media attention, the numbers of male athletes who commit IPV are not significantly higher than males in the general population. And current studies indicate that a male athlete is more likely to become violent in an intimate relationship than a male nonathlete. Nonetheless, when examining the perpetration of IPV among athletes, many experts point to the competitive, macho, and often violent nature of many sports as a "cultivator of aggression." Interestingly, some prevailing theories assert that the same qualities that make for a good athlete can conversely lead to a dysfunctional homelife and IPV [9].

It should be noted that research findings with regard to sports culture and IPV are complicated by inherent challenges in the study of this knotty and complex biopsychosocial issue. In addition to poorly designed studies and scant available research literature, there is rampant inconsistency in use of terminology, the "measurement" of what is considered violent behavior, accurate quantification of relationship dynamics, and failure to take into account the cultural dynamics and context given for survey questions. Accordingly, an in-depth, evidence-based discussion of the multitude of available causative and correlative factors as well as copious ideological and theoretical constructs underpinning the understanding of IPV within sports culture is beyond our scope. The central aim of this chapter is to meaningfully contribute to the IPV and sports culture conversation through a deconstruction of the above case illustration. The unique characteristics associated with the occurrence of IPV among elite male athletes will be explored.

Introduction

It is surmised that IPV among professional male athletes continues to reflect larger, underlying and enduring societal themes. Male privilege, for example, sets sociocultural norms and expectations that inform the notions of power and control that can easily be identified in sports culture. Power and control are at the heart of IPV as well.

Selective media coverage and media bias (i.e., minimizing domestic violence as "domestic disputes") is another example of how larger societal forces contribute to the perpetuation of IPV. Failure of the justice system interventions to generate strong or consistent evidence of deterrent effects on either repeat victimization or repeat offending constitutes yet another overarching and vexing societal problem. It is concluded that sports organizations and professional athletes are uniquely poised to positively influence and advance the movement to eradicate IPV.

Findings about the concerns and challenges of addressing IPV in sports culture are based not only on the analysis of the case illustration but will draw from a review of popular and scholarly IPV literature, interviews with clinical IPV providers, and direct experiences assisting collegiate and professional athletes and their families suffering and coping with IPV.

The Role of Identity and Injury in the Male Athlete with Violent Behaviors

In deconstructing the above case illustration, it is important to consider the roles of masculine identity and athletic identity and how they informed John's self-perception, expectations, and behaviors, especially with regard to the treatment of women. Defining identity in general is no easy task. Celebrated psychoanalyst Erik Erikson grappled with the definition in his seminal work, *Identity, Youth, and Crisis*:

> So far I have tried out the term 'identity' almost deliberately--I like to think—in many different connotations. At one time it seemed to refer to a conscious sense of individual uniqueness, and at a another to an unconscious striving for continuity of experience, and a third as a solidarity with a group's ideals. [10]

From this three-pronged definition, it can be argued that human beings, in fact, have many different identities that surface at different times in different situations. It is immediately apparent how participation in sports might contribute to the simultaneous consolidation of all three aspects of identity postulated by Erikson. Certainly, John feels a sense of "individual uniqueness" in the role of being "a male" and also being "a star athlete" (and benefits from the power and privileges of each of these roles). Secondly, identity cohesion may be bolstered as he unconsciously strives for "continuity of experience" through participation in his sport. Thirdly, by offering the opportunity for "solidarity with the group's ideals," sport offers John a third identity reinforcing opportunity. While this theoretical conceptualization addresses the male identity formation, it does not contemplate factors contributing to female identity. Thus we have little idea of the contributions to Marcia's identity (from the case illustration above) and run the risk of applying male determinants to her identity or, worse, seeing her as "weak" if she doesn't fit the masculine ideal.

Beyond psychoanalytic theory and definitions, gender bias has practical applications in sport culture vis-a-vis the development of traditional masculine identity. At bottom, Western sport identity resonates with Western culture's traditional notions of the patriarchal ideals for masculinity. Images of masculinity as advertised in the media and portrayed in the movies tend to focus on stoicism, power, control, pain tolerance, toughness, self-sufficiency, physics strength, and sexual potency. Boys feel tremendous pressure to always display gender-appropriate behaviors that measure up to the "man code." Most likely, John, from our case illustration, was taught he would be considered a "loser" or weak if he cried in public, wanted to wear pink, or showed public displays of affection and emotional tenderness. The ultimate blow to masculinity in this construct is to be called "a little girl" or "gay."

Through sport and other social institutors, traditionally negative male characteristics tend to be reinforced over time [11]. Players are extolled for outward displays of masculinity, such as being *tough*, *stoic*, *intimidating*, and showing *killer instinct*. Throwing tantrums is considered a sign of male dominance and passion, whereas females displaying the same behavior are labelled "overly emotional," "histrionic," or "butch"—for trying to be "like a man." At best, such emotional displays from female athletes are considered unbecoming. Men, on the other hand, as part of their identities, are often socialized to adhere to patriarchal codes associated with aggressive behaviors [12], especially if their masculinity is threatened. This mandate for asserting power and control in the face of threats from an opponent is true for male athletes in competitive sports.

From the case illustration, it is not difficult to see that John's masculine identity was deeply influenced by his upbringing as a traditional male in Western culture, amid all of the social pressures and cultural cues to be identified and perceived as a "man." Indeed, John's training started in childhood, well before he got into sports, as he witnessed displays of masculine aggression modeled within his own family by older males. The underlying notions of power and control, imbibed and imprinted on his subconscious through family experience, were perhaps amplified in the context of assuming the "alpha male" role on the team—a role that exalts power and control.

A chink in the "masculine armor" occurred when John lost power and control on the team due to the injury. Sidelined, no longer able to attend practice, no longer able to participate in games, and no longer the focus of attention, John's athletic identity took a huge hit. Like most athletes who face a season ending in injury, John was most likely flooded with a myriad of emotions that had to be suppressed. Being hobbled and sidelined meant he could no longer keep up with the herd much less lead it. And it became harder to exert power, control, and influence on the other players if he was no longer able to play and demonstrate his superior skills as a leader (which is a fairly common experience for an injured athlete in most sports). The loss of athletic function and the leadership role on the team may have created an existential crisis for John whose athletic identity was of paramount importance to his self-esteem and self-worth, because he had so little sense of his identity outside of his athletic identity, he felt lost, and started to become frustrated and despondent. He coped with these negative feelings by using alcohol. Drinking served as trigger to lower his defenses and allowed his frustrations and anger to surface. In a disinhibited state, John increased his risk to become threatening and violent. He would then feel guilty about his threatening and violent behaviors and become more upset with himself. Because he could not escape back to his sport because of the injury, John would feel helpless and hopeless and would start drinking again after a period of abstinence, and his cycle with violence would ensue.

Athletes, like John, are sometimes unaware that they have both a private identity (their deepest beliefs, emotions, values, and wishes that they hide from the public eye) and a public identity (what they project to the outside world and what people see and what they think people see). According to role-identity theory, human beings are predisposed to behave based on their self-perceptions and how they would like to be perceived by others—meaning that both the private and public identities contribute to the self-other experience. Generally, the identity a person deems most important is ranked higher than others. For many athletes, like John, who get overcommitted to an athletic identity early in their childhood (or in their careers), they can get locked in on a unidimensional (athletic) identity and experience "identity foreclosure" and never develop a multidimensional identity capable of adapting to setbacks such as injury or retirement. In essence their private and public identities fuse, which is set up for psychological-emotional problems. In John's case, the inability to cope with his injury in the face of a unidimensional view of his personality spelled trouble and pain for him and his wife. John essentially had no knowledge of who he was outside of his sport and did not know how to be at home and in non-sports-oriented circles. Like most athletes John hid this inadequacy very well until he was no longer able to play.

While this explanation in no way excuses John's violent behaviors, the unpacking of John's negative identity conditioning from upbringing in light of his family history, his overly narrowed focus and attachment to his athletic identity, and his poor coping skills (using alcohol, power, control, intimidation, and violence) are discrete and palpable areas for therapeutic intervention. In addition to helping discover where his identity may have been stunted, appropriate intervention will help John take responsibility for his broader identity as a caring and sensitive man and father, as someone with interests outside of his sport—and most importantly as an enlightened being who values and respects the rights of women and children. Because identity is never static and always growing and changing across the human lifespan, John, if guided to develop a broader sense of identity over time, will now have a new set of coping resources to help him tackle and overcome years of negative reinforcement associated with negative masculine conditioning that contribute to violent behaviors.

The Role of Fame, Favor, and Fortune in the Male Athlete with Violent Behaviors

Undoubtedly, John, in the case illustration above, prior to his injury, enjoyed the benefits of his stardom. When he became injured, the psychological benefits of being an alpha male and the admiration and accolades that came along with his athletic performance stopped. Though he still enjoyed a degree of fame and received well wishes from his fans on the side lines, John was acutely aware that he was no longer a part of the action or the limelight. The fall from fame and favor took its toll on John who, as already discussed, depended on his athletic identity for his self-worth and, at some level, for his sense of masculinity. In this case illustration, John admits to drinking and smoking weed to allegedly cope with his temporary fall from favor and fame. He also admits to becoming physically aggressive and violent while drunk and has pushed his wife on more than one occasion claiming to feel intensely disrespected by her. This sense of humiliation—being "disrespected"—can be tied into his injury state as well. He finds his situation and now his wife to be intolerable. From a purely psychological vantage point, John's ego appears to have suffered a crushing blow which surfaced pathological feelings and distortions within John's psyche. As noted by Gilligan in 2003 [13], among others, violence serves to replace feelings of humiliation with feelings of power and pride—and possibly artificially inflating his self-esteem.

Interestingly, one of John's main concerns, aside from potentially losing his job, is the fear of losing favor with the fans. He stated that he has "millions" of fans depending on him and doesn't want to let them down. This assertion by John merits attention. At face value John appears to care about disappointing his fan base, especially the kids as he suggests, but, at a deeper level, John appears to be more concerned about losing popular appeal and favor in the public eye than in the eyes of his wife and immediate family. What this suggests is that he places a higher value on fame and favor than on the pain and suffering he has caused his wife, Marcia.

John's seeming lack of empathy for Marcia and fear of losing public favor are troubling and perhaps emblematic of a larger societal issue with men who commit IPV being more concerned with the loss of reputation than their harmful actions. Some IPV counselors posit that this lack of empathy signals a narcissistic underbelly that is nurtured in professional athletes. They suggest that male athletes operate above the law and because of their fame do not believe "the rules everyone else has to play by" applies to them. Because such athletes are essentially arrogant and entitled, the argument goes, they do not think there is anything wrong with their violent behaviors and are incapable of ever taking full responsibility for their actions. These athletes, according to many IPV counselors, are perfectly happy to live as frauds—that is, publicly accepting all the benefits of public adoration and celebrity status while privately persisting with shameful and violent behaviors toward their partners—behaviors they would never want to go viral. This double standard in attitude toward IPV appears to favor the famous as indicated by several news articles detailing the historically troubling pattern of top male athletes across all sports being allowed to continue in their roles despite evidence of their involvement (and, in some cases, being charged with IPV). Moreover, there is a troubling perception that the attainment of fame often grants some degree of impunity to athletes who commit IPV. The conviction rate of athletes who commit IPV is lower than the general population. A study that looked at conviction rates in 1995 found that only 31% of accused male athletes were convicted. This is in stark contrast to 77% conviction rate of males in the general public [14].

Other theorists disagree with the view that fame, favor, and fortune cause male athletes to become narcissistic and less empathetic to the victims and survivors of their violent actions. They argue that male athletes do empathize with their abused partners but place a high value on their reputations and feel that they will be unfairly vilified and scapegoated with no chance of restitution precisely because they are famous. They argue that they should not have to lose their "bread and butter" because they have been involved with IPV. Some athletes accused of IPV point to the fact that other men in other fields (some even with a degree of notoriety) are able to keep their employment and make a living despite having been charged with IPV. These athletes believe that it is unfair to not allow them an opportunity to rehabilitate. They say it is unfair that some women get to instigate and commit violent acts toward men, but when they try to register a complaint, they are looked as "less than masculine" and laughed at because of their size and muscularity. They consider this a form of reverse discrimination, double standards, and a form of female privilege. Some complain that women have set them up, lied, and claimed violence and were given the benefit of the doubt—and the same courtesy is not afforded to men.

Behind closed counseling doors, some male athletes point to the fact that women change their minds and recant their stories with little to no legal consequences which indicates that men are always "guilty" even if the woman says she lied about the allegations of violence. Others express frustration over the broad reach of IPV that allows someone to be accused of IPV and have to fight the label of being "violent" even if they have not committed an actual violent act. In many cases, they argue, any woman can simply claim to be "feeling threatened or unsafe," which is enough. Male athletes contend that women who are aware of their celebrity status and know the vulnerability associated with an athlete's fame and fortune are quick to take advantage of the broad IPV definition by claiming they feel threatened and unsafe.

In addition to feeling vulnerable to such potential attacks, some male athletes point out that there is basically no bonafide avenue within sports culture, or within society at large, for a man who feels vulnerable to be afforded the benefit of the doubt and granted similar legal protections. Athletes of color express that as "Black men," they are extremely reluctant to engage with law enforcement at any level given the troubled history between Black males and police officers. They argue that if they were to call a police officer to complain about a female threatening them or making them feel unsafe, they would automatically become the suspect—especially if the woman says she felt threatened or unsafe. These athletes believe that there is not only a double standard with respect to men not being allowed to be vulnerable and enjoy the same legal privileges as women with regard to IPV but point out another double IPV standard with regard to how men of color are treated versus the preferential treatment afforded to white males.

Regardless of cultural heritage and the apparent lack of avenues to express their "vulnerability" within the context of IPV, it is not difficult to note that professional male athletes enjoy and benefit from the double privilege of being male and having celebrity status. Athletes have long been revered in American culture—a culture that turns them into heroes. Regardless of their personal backgrounds, beliefs, and volition, these athletes are widely regarded as role models by fans, advertisers, and society at large.

Along with the fame, favor, and fortune come the status and influence of their stardom, which few refuse. Professional athletes, often unwittingly, wear the idealized hero-role-model-expectation mantle not only in the most public performance spheres but in their private lives as well. Some are not fully aware that their success means they must live with additional pressure of intense public scrutiny at all times. After all, the very definition of "role model," according to Webster's dictionary, is "a person whose behavior in a particular role is imitated by others" [15]. A "hero" is defined as "a person admired for achievements and noble qualities. The focus in American culture (and in sports culture) tends to be on the hero's achievements and generally not on character or "noble qualities"—unless and until the "hero" runs into a problem or is the brunt of an accusation.

Blinded by the bright lights of heroic status and stardom, some of these idealized and exalted athletes are broadsided by the precipitous fall from fame and the loss of favor and fortune when implicated in the perpetration of IPV. Behind closed doors, they are often stunned by the massive attention and outrage their actions have precipitated. Beyond drawing national attention, IPV, in the context of a male-dominant sports culture, raises several issues emblematic of a larger societal problem: How societal hero worship in sports cultures contributes to distorted notions of power and control within the construct of masculinity and negatively affects their intimate partner relationships? For some athletes, the intense scrutiny and public expectation appear unrealistic. Charles Barkley drew attention to the complexity of this issue with the forthright statement: "I'm not paid to be a role model. I'm paid to wreak havoc on the basketball court" [16]. Barkley's observation was immortalized in a widely seen television commercial that stirred the debate on the role of athletes within American culture. What remains undebatable is that fame, fortune, and favor will always carry with them a level of scrutiny that will always draw public attention to the "good" and the "bad" that athletes do. Moreover, fame and fortune do not exonerate perpetrators of violence but in fact holds them more accountable in the court of public perception and opinion. In light of the recent national attention paid to IPV, most sports organizations provide awareness and sensitivity training to help athletes understand the hidden expectations and potential pitfalls that come along with fame, favor, and fortune. It is surmised that this is a positive and important step that should be supplemented with ongoing IPV sensitivity training. A number of sports organizations are now implementing these trainings.

Why Do Women Involved with Athletes Accused of IPV Stay?

In the case illustration above, Marcia displayed a pattern of justification, vacillation, and ambivalence that is fairly typical of women trapped in the IPV cycle. Marcia, who clearly loves John, attempts to minimize the magnitude of her situation by claiming that she is not negatively affected by John's behaviors. She feels this way because she is accustomed to seeing men act violently toward women having grown up in such a household. It is possible that Marcia may have been desensitized by her childhood and past experiences or she may be attempting to keep the peace at home and cope with John's behaviors because she sees little hope of John ever changing.

Another mitigating factor in her decision to stay with John is Marcia's belief that the good news of her pregnancy will positively affect John's psyche and thereby reduce his violent tendencies. Although the research data on the prevalence of IPV during pregnancy are equivocal, with some studies showing a lower rate of occurrence, it remains clear that women who experience IPV during pregnancy are at higher risk for negative outcomes, including low birthweight and preterm pregnancy [17]. Interestingly, while IPV can be found among partners from all socioeconomic levels, a number of studies have suggested certain women may be at increased risk of IPV during pregnancy due to lower socioeconomic status (SES), age, marital status, or minority status [18, 19].

Marcia indicated she felt a need to protect John and his career and did not want his earning potential as an athlete to suffer. She shared feelings of satisfaction that John had provided her with a lifestyle and assets they had built that she did not want them to lose. Convinced that John would change and that she did not need help, Marcia never engaged in therapeutic intervention. For a brief period, the relationship between Marcia and John appeared to have improved. But, as is too often the case with IPV, the cycle resurfaced, and Marcia filed an Order of Protection against John, which she later attempted to rescind.

There is very little evidence-based research in the IPV literature addressing the reasons women who are married to elite athletes choose to stay in violent relationships. It is surmised that they stay for the same reasons women trapped in the cycle of IPV choose to remain. In the case of women who are in a relationship with a sports figure, there is the added burden of having to navigate his public persona along with the power and status it carries. In a world of male privilege, sports figures arguably enjoy and wield tremendous power and influence which could potentially make their partners reluctant and incapable of going up against them. Some women have confided that they were afraid of the backlash from avid fans and organizations that revere their husbands. Some worried that they would be perceived as opportunists. Others feared that they would be criticized for waiting "too long" before speaking up. Like Marcia, some women feared that they would lose the lifestyle they had become accustomed to. Others indicated that they felt guilty about complaining because their husbands would lavish them with such expensive gifts after a violent outburst and they would "feel bad" about speaking out. Several women shared that speaking out and speaking up only made the likelihood of physical retaliation worse and that having a powerful sports figure as a partner put additional pressure on them to stay quiet so that they would not have to endure the spectacle of being in the news and on social media.

According to the National Center on Domestic Violence, Trauma & Mental Health [20], the motivations and experiences of women who dare to come forward are always questioned and placed under far more scrutiny than the men they accuse, even when making these accusations gets them nothing in return. Small wonder that women are reluctant to engage and trust the system. Based on this observation, some prosecutors approach IPV cases like homicide cases with the assumption that there will be no victim to testify. Many IPV advocates and legal experts agree that women are often in a no-win situation when they come forward as accusers. For example, the celebrated case of Amber Heard and the restraining order she filed against her husband, Johnny Depp, stating that he'd been emotionally and physically abusive toward her for much of their marriage was received with criticism [21]. Some people have been publicly skeptical of Amber because she has a successful career and is financially independent. They argue that Amber had "no reason not to leave a violent situation." Ultimately this speaks to the lack of comprehension of all the factors that contribute to a woman's reluctance to immediately leave a violent relationship, after having invested her heart, life, love, and soul. In this case, Amber's financial success and status were used as evidence that she is, in fact, "lying about the whole thing." Amber's outcome speaks to the vexing theme that financial insecurity is the *only reason* someone would stay in such a situation.

Ultimately, women who love partners that commit IPV are automatically put into an extremely complex and potentially life-altering situation. Being attached to a partner who is publicly honored and idealized but who is controlling and violent in the privacy of the home creates a delicate situation. Many of the partners of male athletes have signed prenuptial agreements, do not work, and are not financially independent. Some are mothers of the household; and others have given up their lives to live on the road or in different cities to provide support to the athlete. Women of famous partners may suffer from lowered self-worth and self-esteem after years of being in the shadow of their famous partners. This low self-esteem is further damaged by the violence and hurts their capacity to be emotionally strong enough to make radical, life-altering decisions. Many may genuinely love their partners and remain forever hopeful because they know a more loving and gentle side of him. As stated before, their situation is different from the general public because of the media frenzy that usually ensues once word of the violence gets out. These are just some of the variables that women must skillfully navigate as they contemplate leaving the home, caring for themselves and finding a new home and reality for themselves and their children, and breaking off the relationship with their partners. It is not surprising that in our case illustration, Marcia decided to stick with John even after filing charges and taking out an Order of Protection.

Are Professional Sports Organizations and Athletes Involved in IPV?

As stated at the outset of this chapter, IPV is technically not a sports culture problem. It is a much larger public health problem that affects thousands of individuals, regardless of age, economic status, race, religion, ethnicity, sexual orientation, or educational background. The majority of those perpetrating this significant, yet preventable, public health issue are men, some of whom happen to be athletes. To be fair, sports organizations, like many other business organizations, are not set up to tackle a public health issue as large and complex as IPV nor are they especially equipped to assess and identify those at highest risk for being perpetrators. In the case illustration above, John's organization, as is most likely the case for many sports organizations, was not initially aware of his deeper issues with substance use and IPV. They were primarily concerned with the observable changes in emotional well-being, presumably secondary to a serious injury. As with most men in larger society, including places of worship, IPV behaviors are hidden and rarely surface until it has reached a crisis proportion.

Despite the limitations of most sports organizations with regard to addressing the epidemic of IPV, social scientists and domestic violence advocates contend that elite athletes who are guilty of IPV are able to perpetuate their behaviors under the protection (and with the tacit support) of organizations, which do little to nothing to sanction or punish them. Some advocates point out that because sports help to shape male identity—and in some ways promote male aggressiveness, ego, power, dominance, and aggression—sports organizations bear a responsibility to ensure that IPV (and all violence) is wrong and punishable. A cursory glance of the popular literature is littered with articles about star athletes across all major sports not receiving meaningful consequences for perpetrating IPV. Instead, many organizations offer rationalizations and justifications to explain away the behavior of their athletes. Some critics believe sports agencies inability to openly declare war on all forms of domestic violence and failure to take definitive punitive action against IPV perpetrators sends a strong message that winning is more important than the safety and well-being of women—many of whom report that they are not consulted when sports leagues conduct their investigations into alleged IPV by its athletes.

While some organizations have no formal domestic violence policy, many of the majority of the professional sports leagues, including baseball, football, hockey, and basketball, are now mandating domestic violence, sexual assault, and sexual harassment training for all players and in many cases coaches and staff. These leagues, in the wake of high-profile IPV cases involving their athletes, have taken major steps to strengthen their professional conduct policies. They now offer stiffer punitive consequences, including suspensions and expulsions from the league for violent behaviors. The National Football League, Major League Baseball, and the National Basketball Association put into place policies specifically addressing domestic, sexual, and child abuse. All offer therapy and counseling and allow leagues to independently investigate incidents. The NHL, despite not having a formal domestic violence policy like other North American professional sports leagues, says it takes each incident on a case-by-case basis. Recently the NHL, based on its independent investigation, suspended a player for an entire season because of IPV he perpetrated in 2014, even though the charges had been dismissed by the legal system. In commenting about the NHL's decision, the commissioner stated: "Today's ruling, while tailored to the specific facts of this case and the individuals involved, is necessary and consistent with the NHL's strongly-held policy that it cannot and will not tolerate this and similar types of conduct, particularly as directed at a spouse, domestic partner or family member" [22]. In 2018, the Los Angeles Times reported on the NHL taking an unusual step to publicly criticize an arbiter who reduced a suspension the league had imposed on an IPV-involved athlete. The suspension was reduced from 27 regular season games to 18 after the NHL Players' Assn. appealed to a neutral arbitrator. In response the NHL released the following statement: "We have reviewed Arbitrator Shyam Das' opinion in the NHLPA's appeal…and are disappointed with the Arbitrator's decision. We firmly believe that the right of appeal to an arbitrator of League discipline was never intended to substitute the arbitrator's judgment for that of the Commissioner, particularly on matters of important League policy and the articulation of acceptable standards of conduct for individuals involved in the National Hockey League" [23].

Stronger and stricter measures against athletes involved in domestic violence are being enacted at the collegiate level. The Southeastern Conference recently unveiled a new policy disallowing players charged and convicted of IPV from playing on any conference team. Per ESPN.com, the policy states, "a transfer student-athlete who has been subject to official university of athletics department disciplinary action at any time during enrollment at any previous collegiate institution (excluding limited discipline applied by a sports team or temporary disciplinary action during an investigation) due to serious misconduct (as defined herein) shall not be eligible for athletically-related financial aid, practice or competition at an SEC member institution" [24].

As encouraging as the heightened responses by sports leagues may be, the roadblocks and barriers to addressing IPV still present a formidable challenge, especially for athletes in need of rehabilitation. Punishing the IPV athlete with suspensions or expulsions sends an important message to all athletes and to society at large, but it does not truly address this public health problem at its root. Some difficult questions sports organizations face center on how to recognize high-risk males and what are the implications associated with labelling someone "high risk." In our case illustration, John came from a family background significant for IPV, has a history of substance use, and holds traditional gender role beliefs. Does this make him high risk? Should all males who fit this profile be excluded from participation in professional sports? John mentioned not connecting with his therapist believing that the therapist did not understand his unique pressures as an athlete. Should he have been seen by a sports psychologist trained in IPV? Are there sports psychologists with specific training is this area? If so, how accessible are they? If

John were to agree to attend a formal IPV batterers program, where would he, as a star athlete, go to get help? Are there IPV programs set up to meet the specific needs of athletes? If so, how accessible are they? A cursory Google search for such programs was unproductive. If John was never convicted of IPV and there was no witnessing of his behaviors and his wife vouches for him, should he be allowed to resume playing? Where are the success stories of professional athletes who have been effectively rehabbed post-perpetrating IPV? Is there a "cure?" Should wives, in light of their willingness to stay involved with their partners, be trusted to give the green light stating that their partners have been transformed? Should men who commit IPV be allowed to reap the benefits associated with engagement in professional sports? Should the intimate partners (including former lovers) of draft picks be interviewed to help determine the existence of IPV? Obviously answers to these questions are beyond the scope and ambit of this chapter but merit further thought and consideration.

What Does the Future Hold?

Fortunately, John's organization had an on-site sports psychologist who was, at least, able to assess and identify his issue with IPV and offer both John and Marcia therapeutic interventions. But as we can infer from their outcome and from contemplation of the questions above, the practical application of real-time interventions for professional athletes and their loved ones is at best a complex navigation that requires a nuanced understanding of the psychosocial complexities involved in assisting and treating couples locked in an IPV cycle. Helping Marcia achieve safety, though a priority, proved difficult given her understandable reluctance. Assisting John with his substance use, violent behaviors, and coping skills requires more than just individual counseling, but finding an appropriate male batterers' program was difficult, and he would not agree to attend. Forcibly separating John and Marcia was not an option. Mandating that Marcia and John would comply with therapy was not feasible. It is therefore not surprising that many sports organizations, after having imposed penalties and offering counseling to all parties involved, simply wait for the storm of media attention to pass and move on.

In sum, IPV-involved male athletes (and their partners) face a myriad of unique treatment and rehabilitation challenges. It is unclear that current interventions show evidence of meaningful transformation. Intervention at the professional sports level is punitive, which serves as a major deterrent. Though such measures are useful and important, it's unclear that they change negative attitudes toward women and the ensuing violent male behaviors. Education and awareness training at the professional level are indeed important and necessary, but it is also unclear if these activities (which may only happen sporadically in a busy season) actually change entrenched male gender biases or reduce violent behaviors toward women. Regrettably, national research on legal interventions, male batterer interventions, and domestic violence programs suggest that they are minimally helpful in reducing male violence and recidivism. Given these grim outcome realities, it is clear that sports culture will not be able to cure this public health crisis. Nonetheless, it bears a responsibility to not perpetuate these atrocities.

By continuing to use its global platform to publicly renounce all forms of IPV and to educate as well as increase domestic violence training and awareness, especially among young males, sports organizations are uniquely poised to offer a major public service in the ongoing fight to eradicate IPV. Continuing the current trend to hold offending athletes accountable for violent actions above and beyond the legal system and partnering with as well as providing financial support, domestic violence shelters, programs, and initiatives will significantly contribute to eliminating IPV on a larger scale. Lastly, developing appropriate, evidence-based, athlete-specific violence prevention and intervention rehabilitation programs would fill a significant gap in the current treatment-intervention landscape.

References

1. Black MC. Intimate partner violence and adverse health consequences: implications for clinicians. Am J Lifestyle Med. 2011;5(5):428–39.
2. Crofford LJ. Violence, stress, and somatic syndromes. Trauma Violence Abuse. 2007;8(3):299–313.
3. Pico-Alfonso MA. Psychological intimate partner violence: the major predictor of posttraumatic stress disorder in abused women. Neurosci Biobehav Rev. 2005;29(1):181–93.
4. Pico-Alfonso MA, Garcia-Linares MI, Celda-Navarro N, Blasco-Ros C, Echeburúa E, Martinez M. The impact of physical, psychological, and sexual intimate male partner violence on women's mental health: depressive symptoms, posttraumatic stress disorder, state anxiety, and suicide. J Women's Health. 2006;15(5):599–611.
5. Pico-Alfonso MA, Garcia-Linares MI, Celda-Navarro N, Herbert J, Martinez M. Changes in cortisol and dehydroepiandrosterone in women victims of physical and psychological intimate partner violence. Biol Psychiatry. 2004;56(4):233–40.
6. Breiding MJ, Black MC, Ryan GW. Prevalence and risk factors of intimate partner violence in eighteen US states/territories, 2005. Am J Prev Med. 2008;34(2):112–8.
7. Logan TK, Shannon L, Cole J, Swanberg J. Partner stalking and implications for women's employment. J Interpers Violence. 2007;22(3):268–91.
8. Randall T. Domestic violence begets other problems of which physicians must be aware to be effective. JAMA. 1990;264(8):940–4.
9. Standen J. The manly sports: the problematic use of criminal law to regulate sports violence. J Crim L Criminol. 2008;99:619.
10. Erikson E. Youth: identity and crisis. New York: W. W. Norton Company; 1968.
11. Broidy LM, Nagin DS, Tremblay RE, Bates JE, Brame B, Dodge KA, Fergusson D, Horwood JL, Loeber R, Laird R, Lynam DR. Developmental trajectories of childhood disruptive behaviors and adolescent delinquency: a six-site, cross-national study. Dev Psychol. 2003;39(2):222.
12. Levant RF, Cuthbert A, Richmond K, Sellers A, Matveev A, Mitina O, Sokolovsky M, Heesacker M. Masculinity ideology among Russian and US young men and women and its relationships to unhealthy lifestyles habits among young Russian men. Psychol Men Masculinity. 2003;4(1):26.
13. Gilligan J. Shame, guilt, and violence. Soc Res Int Quart. 2003;70(4):1149–80.
14. Benedict J, Klein A. Arrest and conviction rates for athletes accused of sexual assault. Sociol Sport J. 1997;14(1):86–94.
15. Merriam-Webster. https://www.merriam-webster.com/dictionary/role%20model. July 2019.
16. Goldman R, Papson S. Nike culture: the sign of the swoosh, London:SAGE Publications; 1998.

17. Alhusen JL, Ray E, Sharps P, Bullock L. Intimate partner violence during pregnancy: maternal and neonatal outcomes. J Women's Health. 2015;24(1):100–6.
18. Coker AL, Sanderson M, Dong B. Partner violence during pregnancy and risk of adverse pregnancy outcomes. Paediatr Perinat Epidemiol. 2004;18(4):260–9.
19. Dunn LL, Oths KS. Prenatal predictors of intimate partner abuse. J Obstet Gynecol Neonatal Nurs. 2004;33(1):54–63.
20. National Center on Domestic Violence, Trauma & Mental Health. www.nationalcenterdvtraumamh.org. October 2019.
21. Yahr E. Amber Heard files restraining order against Johnny Depp after alleged domestic violence. https://www.washingtonpost.com/news/arts-and-entertainment/wp/2016/05/27/amber-heard-files-restraining-order-against-johnny-depp-after-alleged-domestic-violence/. May 27, 2016.
22. The Los Angeles Times. NHL suspends Kings' Slava Voynov after arrest. https://www.latimes.com/sports/kings/la-sp-kings-voynov-arrest-20141021-story.html. October 21, 2014.
23. The Los Angeles Times. NHL slams arbitrator's decision to reduce domestic violence suspension of Predators' Austin Watson. https://wwwlatimescom/sports/hockey/la-sp-sn-nhl-domestic-violence-20181012-storyhtml. October 12, 2018.
24. Ching D. SEC: schools can't take transfers with serious misconduct past. ESPN. https://www.espn.com/college-football/story/_/id/12977228/sec-adopts-proposal-prevents-transfer-students-histories-domestic-violence-sexual-assault. May 29, 2015.

Violent Childhood: Domestic Violence in Childhood

13

A. Dexter Samuels and Rahn Kennedy Bailey

This book has identified how a wide range of people are affected by violence at the hands of their intimate partner. This chapter will explore the consequences of intimate partner violence (IPV) on another vulnerable population. In the United States, up to ten million children are exposed to IPV in the form of abuse against a parent [1]. Children exposed to IPV have increased mental and physical health consequences. These effects are widespread and observed in children of all ages. Witnessing IPV among one's parents puts children at higher risk of experiencing IPV as adults [1]. Irrespective of cause, exposure to parental depression places children at risk for behavior problems and decreased cognitive performance [1]. In the study, Associations of Early Exposure to Intimate Partner Violence and Parental Depression with Subsequent Mental Health Outcomes, exposure to both IPV and parental depression before age 3 years was associated with preschool-aged onset of ADHD [1].

It has been observed that children whose parents suffer from IPV are at increased risk for onset of ADHD during preschool. Evidence shows school-aged children experiencing parental IPV have more academic difficulties when compared to children not experiencing IPV. Academic problems can be low grades, poor school attendance, and grade repetition [2].

Children in households where IPV occurs are more likely to have nurse visits resulting in the child being sent home [2]. Additionally, children who experience parental intimate partner violence suffer from speech pathology at higher rates than nonexposed children [2].

A. D. Samuels
Center for Health Policy, Meharry Medical College, Nashville, TN, USA

R. K. Bailey (✉)
Department of Psychiatry, Charles R. Drew University of Medicine and Science, Los Angeles, CA, USA
e-mail: rahnkbaileymd@comcast.net

R. K. Bailey (ed.), *Intimate Partner Violence*,
https://doi.org/10.1007/978-3-030-55864-2_13

As mentioned earlier in this book, experiencing IPV can send a victim into depression. If that victim is a parent, then the debilitating effects of the disease (depression) can undoubtedly diminish the quality of their ability to deliver child care. Indeed, even the youngest of children can be negatively affected by IPV. Mothers who suffer from abuse tend to have children of lower weight, who exhibit less weight gain, and more irritability [2]. It has been proposed that this trend may be a result of the traumatic effects of abuse reducing the mother's ability to acutely care for the child after an episode of abuse. IPV, depression, and substance abuse have all been shown to reduce maternal functioning [3]. Therefore, no child is too young to be impacted by parental IPV.

Sadly, factors that reduce the quality of maternal functioning and caretaking tend to cluster together. That is to say, women experiencing IPV are at increased risk for depression and substance abuse. This negatively impacts the quality of care they can deliver and places children at higher risk for developmental disorders [4].

Care must be taken to identify children who experience parental IPV. Experiencing violence occurring among adults can be very frightening for a child. This effect is likely magnified when the violence is inflicted on a parent. Moreover, it is known that a victim of IPV lives in a state of fear and constant distress. Likely, this stress burdens a child whose domestic environment includes IPV. Repeated or graphic exposures to such trauma can lead to difficulty adjusting. Between 17% and 33% of school-aged children meet clinical criteria for post-traumatic stress disorder (PTSD) [5]. PTSD in young children can manifest as clinginess, talking or thinking about the event repeatedly, and recurrent nightmares. In addition, a child who lives in a household where IPV occurs is more likely to experience other forms of interpersonal trauma. Interpersonal trauma can be events such as child abuse, sexual abuse, or assault. Children are 2.5 times more likely to be physically abused and almost 5 times more likely to be sexually abused than are children living in a home without IPV [5].

There are established negative consequences for children who experience parental IPV. If IPV is not considered a form of child abuse in a jurisdiction, the perpetrator's access to children is not limited. As discussed throughout this book, a victim's relationship with their abuser is complex. A parent's relationship with an abuser can be protracted. Victims often return to the perpetrator of abuse repeatedly before the relationship is permanently terminated. Additionally, children could possibly experience other disruptions in their environment such as homelessness or assignment to a shelter. Often the victim weighs options considering what would be best for the child. Especially with younger kids, it may be assumed that the young child is oblivious to the ongoing parental violence.

However, children are often aware of the abuse. During times of abuse, be it yelling or physical violence, children are frightened. They may feel as though they are the source of the conflict. Many women with children who have left their abuser have cited their child being injured, remarking about the abuse, or mimicking the abuser behavior as reasons for leaving.

Other negative health consequences have been seen in children whose parent is a victim of IPV.

Obesity is a growing public health concern. Obese children are more likely to be obese in adulthood [6]. The health risks associated with obesity have been well-documented. Some risks to health include higher risks for hypertension, high cholesterol, diabetes, heart disease, stroke, and cancer [6]. Obesity in children has been largely attributed to family environment. Mostly, the typical reasons given have been sedentary lifestyle and an excess of calorie-rich foods. However, little has been done to explore the psychological factors that influence both the child and caregiver on food choices.

An association between obesity in children and IPV has been established. 80% of children, whose mothers experienced chronic IPV, were reported to be obese by age 5 [6]. There is some speculation as to the cause of this phenomenon, and a few explanations have been put forth. How a mother feeds her child may be influenced by IPV. This may lead to food being used as a consolation tool by the mother. Additionally, it is thought children may intake more calorie-rich food as a way to self-soothe [6].

Living in a household where parental IPV occurs can subject children to tremendous psychological stress. This increased stress burden can manifest in the form of physical illness. It is thought that stress exposure during infancy and early childhood exaggerates some physiological systems responses to stress [7]. This disruption of stress regulation has been linked to asthma [7]. Moreover, a child's ability to cope effectively with stress may be formed in the context of a good mother-child relationship. That is to say, insensitive maternal attentiveness to a stressed child may disrupt that child's neuroimmune development, setting the stage for asthma [7]. This reinforces the importance of a caregiver's ability to tend to a child appropriately. Maternal IPV victimization and its deleterious effect on a child's caregiver (the mother) can reduce the quality of child rearing and so lead to poor stress regulation in the child. This is a less intuitive example of how maternal IPV victimization can lead to poorer health in a child.

Adverse health conditions are seen in children exposed to IPV. There is an increased risk for asthma in early childhood. There has been growing evidence linking stress to childhood asthma. Stress during infancy and early childhood may have complex neurobiological consequences. Disrupted patterns in stress regulation and its interplay immune system are thought to put IPV children at a higher risk of asthma [7]. A child's ability to cope (self-regulate) with stress is thought to be a reflection of the child and the caregiver's early relationship.

Self-regulation is the ability to modulate one's outward emotional state and behavior in a social setting. Children with good adaptive behavior and coping mechanisms tend to also have good self-regulation. A good caregiver relationship helps foster self-regulation in a child. This milestone of self-regulation is usually reached at the preschool age. It is thought that having an insensitive or unemotionally engaged caregiver leads to underdeveloped self-regulation leading to maladaptive behavior and disrupts the neuroimmune pathways causing greater risk of asthma.

Children with asthma have been shown to have higher degrees of emotional deregulation [7]. This emphasizes the importance of the caregiver in influencing both the emotional and physical health of a child. IPV violence causes a reduction in the ability of a person to give adequate care and attention to a child. This reduction in the quality of care a child receives can in turn lead to a poor nutritional or behavioral state.

Efforts have been made to predict and prevent IPV in children. Some observable predictors of perpetrating IPV later in life have been identified. Children exposed to parental intimate partner violence and child abuse (physical or sexual) have an increased likelihood of perpetrating IPV as adults. The sex of the child plays a predictive role as well. The overwhelming majority of IPV perpetrators are male. 20–40% of adult males have perpetrated IPV at some point [8].

Violence Perpetration Some studies point to frequent bullying of other children as a good predictor of future IPV [8]. As discussed throughout this book, there is a typical pattern of behavior displayed by perpetrators of abuse. It is thought that the same impulses that lead a person to bully as a child may also lead them to commit violence against an intimate partner in the future. It is thought that both patterns of behavior stem from a desire to control and coerce someone who is perceived to be weaker [8].

Witnesses of parental IPV have immediate and long-term physical and psychological health consequences. Additionally, children in a household where parental IPV occurs are more likely to be the next generation of victims or perpetrators [9]. Indeed, witnessing IPV puts a child at higher risk for being a victim of IPV later in life. This is particularly true for female children. It is thought that violence is normalized among children who have witnessed parental IPV. Violence may be viewed as a normal way that conflict and disagreement are solved. Interestingly, 56% of abused mothers have reported that their children did not witness IPV that had occurred. Though the child may not have witnessed the violent act, they may still be aware of the ongoing violence [9], thus possibly exposing them to potential additional stress and/or normalization of domestic violence.

IPV is an established concern seen among adult women. Sadly, the trend of violence against partners is seen among adolescents as well. Just as intimate partner violence is a major concern regarding adult women, adolescent girls suffer from IPV at rates similar to the adult population. IPV puts adolescent girls at risk for other behaviors that have negative impacts on their health. These behaviors can be substance abuse risk and unhealthy body weight regulation (diet pill, laxative use, vomiting). Adolescent girls experiencing IPV are more likely to have had three or more sexual partners in the last 3 months. Adolescents experiencing IPV or dating violence are less likely to have used condoms during their last sexual encounter. This puts them at higher risk for STI and teen pregnancy. Additionally, this group has exhibited higher serious contemplations of suicide or attempts at suicide. About 10% of intentional injuries to adolescent girls are reportedly inflicted by a male they were dating [10].

Dating violence is pervasive among both boys and girls. Most adolescents seen in an emergency room setting have reported experiencing violence with a person they were dating. This particular study showed higher female perpetrators of violence [11]. However, more severe forms of dating violence were perpetrated by males. Furthermore, female victims were more likely to report being afraid of being injured by their partner. This further substantiates that girls are more likely to have greater health risks while in a relationship with partner violence. Adolescents tend to experience a higher rate of mutual IPV [11].

Among males, perpetrating bullying of others suggested possible perpetration of IPV as an adult. Among adolescent females, those with depressive symptoms were shown to be more likely to be the victim of abuse. Depressive symptoms of low self-esteem, low satisfaction, and internalization are occurring at a time when young females are gaining more independence. It is thought that their psychological vulnerability at this age leads to riskier behavior and association with others who also partake in risky behavior. Additionally, males with depressive symptoms tend to use aggression against an intimate partner [12]. Moreover, a depressed female may be less likely to leave. During the depressed period, she may have achieved low education and be more financially tied to the abuser and have less robust support from friends and family.

Thankfully, some efforts have been made to proactively prevent dating violence. Programs to educate high school students about healthy relationships, sexual health, and substance use prevention have been implemented. Among teens who received IPV education in school, IPV and substance abuse were observed to be reduced in this group upon 2.5 year follow-up (compared with teens who did not receive this educational intervention) [13].

In this chapter, we have seen the far-reaching effects of IPV on children. It is important to note that a child of any age can suffer from parental intimate partner violence. Women in an abusive relationship often are solely responsible for child rearing. Abuse and the associated isolation that is common in IPV relationships often overburden a caretaker and diminish their parental care. Despite earnest attempts, it is exceedingly hard to shield a child from abuse that occurs at home. This stress component can lead to maladaptive behaviors in children and predispose them to a variety of medical and mental health issues. Children in a home routinely perform worse in school and receive more disciplinary action.

Children who are witness to IPV are more likely to be absent from school. Absenteeism often is due to an illness that likely has stress-induced component. However, there are heartbreaking stories of children electing to stay home in the hopes of protecting the abused parent. Sadly, children may be inadvertently hurt during an episode of IPV occurring at home. This can be exceedingly burdensome for mothers who may feel a sense of failure for not protecting their children. However, it has been noted that a child's well-being has often been the critical factor for abused mothers in deciding to leave or stay in an abusive relationship. Some promise has been shown regarding school and behavior improvement in children who have been removed from an environment where IPV was occurring.

Witnessing the abuse of a parent predisposes a child to either be the perpetrator or victim of abuse later in adult life. Some studies suggest that bullying is a predictive factor in boys perpetrating partner violence as men. Conversely, the likelihood of being a victim was associated with depression in adolescent females. The increased observed risk for abuse is likely due to risky behavior patterns, peer association, and dating choices that are typically made by depressed teens. Intervention has shown promise in reducing the incidence of IPV. Education regarding healthy relationships, effective communication, and substance abuse avoidance has reduced the cases of violence. This chapter has again emphasized the scope of IPV and the sad reality that children are often collateral damage.

References

1. Bauer NS, Gilbert AL, Carroll AE, Downs SM. Associations of early exposure to intimate partner violence and parental depression with subsequent mental health outcomes. JAMA Pediatr. 2013;167(4):341–7.
2. Kernic MA, Holt VL, Wolf ME, McKnight B, Huebner CE, Rivara FP. Academic and school health issues among children exposed to maternal intimate partner abuse. Arch Pediatr Adolesc Med. 2002;156(6):549–55.
3. McFarlane JM, Groff JY, O'Brien JA, Watson K. Behaviors of children who are exposed and not exposed to intimate partner violence: an analysis of 330 black, white, and Hispanic children. Pediatrics. 2003;112(3):e202–7.
4. Holmes MR. Aggressive behavior of children exposed to intimate partner violence: an examination of maternal mental health, maternal warmth and child maltreatment. Child Abuse Negl. 2013;37(8):520–30.
5. Graham-Bermann SA, Castor LE, Miller LE, Howell KH. The impact of intimate partner violence and additional traumatic events on trauma symptoms and PTSD in preschool-aged children. J Traumatic Stress. 2012;25(4):393–400.
6. Boynton-Jarrett R, Fargnoli J, Suglia SF, Zuckerman B, Wright RJ. Association between maternal intimate partner violence and incident obesity in preschool-aged children: results from the fragile families and child Well-being study. Arch Pediatr Adolesc Med. 2010;164(6):540–6.
7. Suglia SF, Enlow MB, Kullowatz A, Wright RJ. Maternal intimate partner violence and increased asthma incidence in children: buffering effects of supportive caregiving. Arch Pediatr Adolesc Med. 2009;163(3):244–50.
8. Falb KL, McCauley HL, Decker MR, Gupta J, Raj A, Silverman JG. School bullying perpetration and other childhood risk factors as predictors of adult intimate partner violence perpetration. Arch Pediatr Adolesc Med. 2011;165(10):890–4.
9. Cannon EA, Bonomi AE, Anderson ML, Rivara FP. The intergenerational transmission of witnessing intimate partner violence. Arch Pediatr Adolesc Med. 2009;163(8):706–8.
10. Silverman JG, Raj A, Mucci LA, Hathaway JE. Dating violence against adolescent girls and associated substance use, unhealthy weight control, sexual risk behavior, pregnancy, and suicidality. JAMA. 2001;286(5):572–9.
11. Carroll BC, Raj A, Noel SE, Bauchner H. Dating violence among adolescents presenting to a pediatric emergency department. Arch Pediatr Adolesc Med. 2011;165(12):1101–6.
12. Lehrer JA, Buka S, Gortmaker S, Shrier LA. Depressive symptomatology as a predictor of exposure to intimate partner violence among US female adolescents and young adults. Arch Pediatr Adolesc Med. 2006;160(3):270–6.
13. Wolfe DA, Crooks C, Jaffe P, Chiodo D, Hughes R, Ellis W, Stitt L, Donner A. A school-based program to prevent adolescent dating violence: a cluster randomized trial. Arch Pediatr Adolesc Med. 2009;163(8):692–9.

14 Teen Dating Violence

Tiffani L. Bell and Rahn Kennedy Bailey

In addition to the effects of intimate partner violence (IPV) on the lives of children, it often has a seemingly unavoidable downstream impact in the dating lives of adolescents. Therefore, it is particularly important to address the prevalence of teen dating violence (TDV) and its impact on current and future intimate relationships.

When interacting with adolescents in a medical setting, it is important to realize that the adolescent may not be there of her own free will. There may be an aspect of distrust or fear of disclosing sensitive topics. During assessment, a great deal of the appointment is often spent building rapport and proving oneself to be trustworthy of such private information as drug use, sexual orientation, previous sexual encounters, and, if present, dating violence. Teens are often fearful that information shared with the physician or mental health professional will be shared with their parents or guardians, and this could lead to decreased transparency in communication.

As mentioned previously, children and adolescents who have witnessed IPV and violence in the home are more likely to have depression, substance abuse, and personal experiences of IPV in adult relationships. Research has shown that the impact of observed IPV on romantic relationships can affect adolescents as young as 13 years old. 13% of males and 20% of females have been the aggressor in teen dating violence between the ages of 13–16 [1]. It is clear that raising awareness of the possibility of teen dating violence prior to its onset is a priority in preventing patterns that may ultimately continue into the future. The CDC reported in 2019 that TDV affects millions of teens in the United States each year. "1 in 11 female and 1 in 15 male high school students experienced physical dating violence in the last year. 1 in

T. L. Bell
Wake Forest School of Medicine, Department of Child and Adolescent Psychiatry, Winston-Salem, NC, USA

R. K. Bailey (✉)
Department of Psychiatry, Charles R. Drew University of Medicine and Science, Los Angeles, CA, USA
e-mail: rahnkbaileymd@comcast.net

R. K. Bailey (ed.), *Intimate Partner Violence*,
https://doi.org/10.1007/978-3-030-55864-2_14

9 female and 1 in 36 male high school students report experiencing sexual dating violence in the last year" [2].

The Centers for Disease Control and Prevention states that teen dating violence includes "four types of behavior: 1. physical violence--which includes hitting, kicking, or attempts to hurt the partner; 2. sexual violence–forcing a partner to participate in an unwanted sexual activity which could even include non-physical sexual behaviors like sending sexual text messages (sexting) or sending naked pictures; 3. psychological aggression-using non-verbal or verbal comments to exert control over someone; and 4. Stalking--repeated undesired attention that makes the partner feel unsafe [2]."

Teen dating violence can lead to depression, anxiety, substance abuse, truancy, dropping out of school, risky sexual behavior, becoming a perpetrator of TDV, difficulties with future relationships, and suicidal thoughts [3]. It was discovered that older adolescents who experienced TDV were 2.5–4 times more likely to smoke cigarettes, use illicit substances, and drink alcohol than those who were not victims of these violent acts [4].

Early romantic relationships often set the stage for and model future romantic relationships. Adolescence is a time for self-exploration and learning healthy ways to communicate. According to Eric Erikson [5], one of the main goals of adolescence is to figure out what one "stands for," what is most important, and to answer the all-important question of "who am I?" Some teens experience the unfortunate reality of thinking that mistreatment is "normal." When teens grow up in violent households, they may believe that violence is a normal way to resolve conflicts. These teens are less likely to report abuse or mistreatment in their relationships and more likely to allow it to continue until it becomes more severe.

As mentioned previously, acceptance and perception of teen dating violence are important. It is known that childhood exposure to violence and being accepting of violence in general increases the risk of being in a relationship with teen dating violence [6]. Those who have been in previously violent relationships are more likely to accept future violent relationships according to Price and Byers [7].

There is some controversy regarding what groups of people TDV affects most frequently. It is thought that it may disproportionately affect sexual, racial, and ethnic minorities more often.

In fact, teen dating violence has become so prevalent that an intervention developed by the CDC, Dating Matters®: Strategies to Promote Healthy Teen Relationships, was created to target children and adolescents ages 11–14 to prevent TDV before it starts [8]. While that may seem young to some, given the potentially chaotic and violent homes where some children are reared, it is vital to begin broaching this subject sooner rather than later. Addressing the effects of IPV and TDV in our vulnerable children and adolescents will hopefully decrease the impact of IPV in adult relationships. As a result, we may spare future generations from the psychological harm that comes from such violence during these important developmental years.

See Fig. 14.1 below from the CDC for more ways to impact and prevent TDV [2].

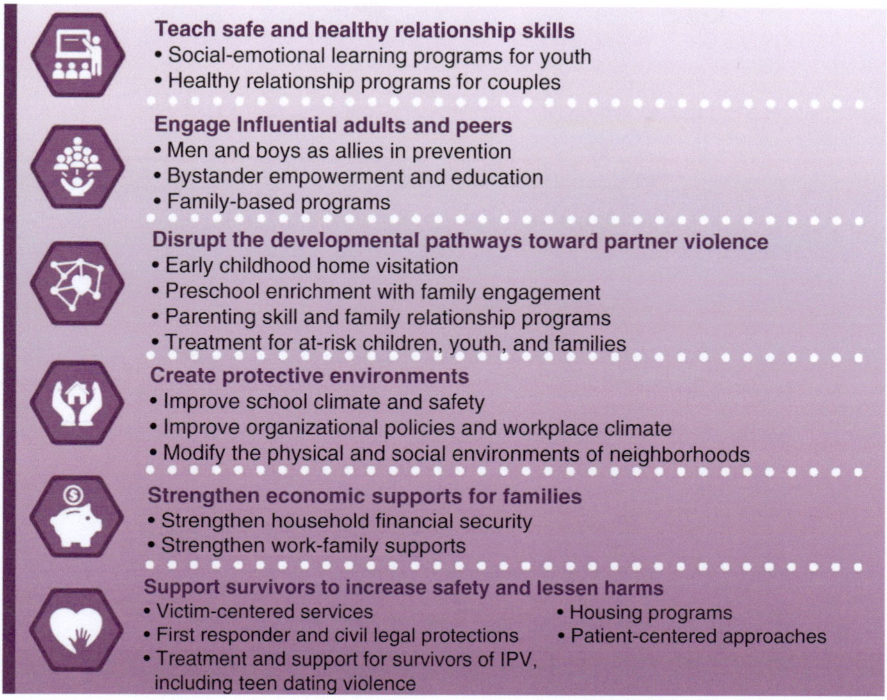
Teach safe and healthy relationship skills
• Social-emotional learning programs for youth
• Healthy relationship programs for couples
Engage Influential adults and peers
• Men and boys as allies in prevention
• Bystander empowerment and education
• Family-based programs
Disrupt the developmental pathways toward partner violence
• Early childhood home visitation
• Preschool enrichment with family engagement
• Parenting skill and family relationship programs
• Treatment for at-risk children, youth, and families
Create protective environments
• Improve school climate and safety
• Improve organizational policies and workplace climate
• Modify the physical and social environments of neighborhoods
Strengthen economic supports for families
• Strengthen household financial security
• Strengthen work-family supports
Support survivors to increase safety and lessen harms
• Victim-centered services
• First responder and civil legal protections
• Treatment and support for survivors of IPV, including teen dating violence
• Housing programs
• Patient-centered approaches

Fig. 14.1 Preventing teen dating violence. (Reprinted from Preventing Teen Dating Violence |Violence Prevention|Injury Center|CDC [2])

References

1. Johnson WL, Giordano PC, Manning WD, Longmore MA. The age–IPV curve: changes in the perpetration of intimate partner violence during adolescence and young adulthood. J Youth Adolesc. 2015;44(3):708–26. https://doi.org/10.1007/s10964-014-0158-z.
2. Preventing Teen Dating Violence |Violence Prevention|Injury Center|CDC. (2019, March 12). Retrieved April 29, 2019, from https://www.cdc.gov/violenceprevention/intimatepartnerviolence/teendatingviolence/fastfact.html.
3. Greenman SJ, Matsuda M. From early dating violence to adult intimate partner violence: continuity and sources of resilience in adulthood. Crim Behav Ment Health. 2016;26(4):293–303. https://doi.org/10.1002/cbm.2012.
4. Temple JR, Freeman DH Jr. Dating violence and substance use among ethnically diverse adolescents. J Interpers Violence. 2011;26(4):701–18. https://doi.org/10.1177/0886260510365858.
5. Rageliene T. Links of adolescence identity development and relationship with peers: a systematic literature review. J Can Acad Child Adolesc Psychiatr. 2016;25(2):97–105.
6. Duke NN, Pettingell SL, McMorris BJ, Borowsky IW. Adolescent violence perpetration: associations with multiple types of adverse childhood experiences. Pediatrics. 2010;125(4):e778–86. https://doi.org/10.1542/peds.2009-0597.
7. Price EL, Byers ES. Attitudes towards dating violence scales. J Family Viol. 1999;14(4):351–75.
8. Dating Matters: Strategies to Promote Healthy Teen Relationships. CDC. https://vetoviolence.cdc.gov/apps/dating-matters-toolkit/.

Intimate Partner Homicide: Firearms Use in Domestic Violence

15

Mohayed Mohayed and Rahn Kennedy Bailey

Intimate partner violence (IPV) is used to control and intimidate victims [1]. The use of violence can often be extreme. Intimate partner assaults involving a firearm are 3 times more likely than those involving a knife [2].

Some violent relationships only terminate with the death of a partner. 1270 intimate partner homicides occurred in 2013 [3]. Of these homicides, about 50% involved the use of a firearm [3]. Additionally, firearms can be used to maintain coercive control in abusive relationships. Intimidation, menace, and power are quickly imbued to most who brandish a firearm. This is seen in the use of firearms in the 32,900 annual occurrences of nonfatal IPV victimizations from 2003 through 2012 [3]. Firearms are the most common weapon used in intimate partner homicides. In 2013, 53% of female intimate partner homicide victims were killed by firearms. In that same year, 40% of male victims were killed by firearms [3]. Knives were the next most commonly used weapon in intimate partner homicide. However, the use of knives yields a more skewed proportion. 19% of women met their demise by knife, while 38% (nearly double) of men were dispatched by knife [3]. Indeed, firearms are not the only method used in IPV. However, it is important to reiterate that they are the leading method.

When guns are restricted, does it influence intimate partner homicide in a meaningful way? About 3.5 people are killed in the United States everyday by their intimate partner. This constitutes a staggering one-third of female homicide victims (killed by a current or former intimate partner) [3].

It is true that the damage from IPV is expansive, can be physical, psychological, and emotional, and does not always involve a gun.

M. Mohayed
Charles R. Drew University College of Medicine, Los Angeles, CA, USA

R. K. Bailey (✉)
Department of Psychiatry, Charles R. Drew University of Medicine and Science, Los Angeles, CA, USA
e-mail: rahnkbaileymd@comcast.net

R. K. Bailey (ed.), *Intimate Partner Violence*,
https://doi.org/10.1007/978-3-030-55864-2_15

However, the mere presence of a firearm in the home may serve in itself as an implicit threat to victims. Additionally, if the nature of violence escalates, a firearm is an exceedingly efficient lethal tool to have at hand. Indeed, assaults involving firearms were significantly more likely to result in death than assaults involving knives or bodily force [3].

Fortunately, the rates of intimate partner homicides have fallen since times past. There was a fall of 50% between 1982 and 2002 [3]. Some have attributed this fall to the following:

- Long-term declines in marriage rates
- Increasing age of first marriage
- Decreased economic dependence of women on men
- Increased availability of services for victims of domestic violence [3]

Furthermore, there have been laws instituted that have limited the access to guns for individuals with a current restraining order against them or with a domestic violence-related conviction [4]. There have been state and federal laws that restrict gun ownership. The Federal Gun Control Act, passed as a part of the Violent Crime Control Act in 1994, was one. The act made it a federal crime to be in possession of a firearm while under a restraining order protecting an intimate partner or their child [4].

An amendment was later added in 1996. This amendment created a second portion to the law. Commonly known as the Lautenberg Amendment, this statute prohibits possession or receipt of a firearm by anyone who has ever been convicted of a qualifying misdemeanor crime of domestic violence [5].

States have a variety of laws regarding the ability of law enforcement officers to confiscate firearms at the scene/home where a domestic violence incident is being investigated.

Women are nine times as likely to be killed by an intimate partner (husband, boyfriend, same-sex partner, or ex) than by a stranger [6]. There have been changes put forth by the justice department that correspond to the decrease in intimate partner homicides over the past three decades [7]. These changes involve better training for law enforcement, increased penalties for domestic violence perpetration, and increased advocacy. Domestic violence hotlines have been created along with women's shelters. Additionally, IPV and its ill-effects on children have come to light during this time. IPV support has now been recognized as a component to child safety. Thus, many child welfare programs are beginning to work hand in hand with domestic violence advocacy organizations [8].

Close examination shows that the group with the largest benefit from the decrease in intimate partner homicide has been men. Increased social awareness and advocacy programs have given women who may be economically dependent ways to escape their abusive partner. Thus, the last resort effort of slaying their intimate partner is not as often reached by women. Compared to years past, women are more aware of the available options regarding refuge from abuse. This has lead Campbell et al. to note, "Homicides by female intimate partners has decreased and the proportion of femicides (murder of women) by male intimate partners has increased" [8].

The best predictor regarding intimate partner homicide (so far) has been previous intimate partner violence in that relationship. 67% to 75% of intimate partner homicides happen in the context of reported histories of intimate partner violence. This is irrespective of which partner is ultimately killed.

In conclusion, IPV in all its various forms can be a terrifying ordeal for victims. The intensity of dread and helplessness that a victim of abuse experiences can often be amplified when their life is threatened. These types of threats are made graver when firearms are involved. In the United States, 30% of murdered women were killed by an intimate partner [8]. Most (55%) were committed using a firearm [9]. Therefore, efforts intended to increase women's safety should be directed at examining domestic partner dynamics. The mere ownership of firearms is a risk factor for intimate partner homicide [10, 11]. Firearms are used in the majority of intimate partner homicides [12, 13, 14, 15]. Ironically, advocacy, and awareness have reduced the rate of male intimate partner homicide victims. Women now have more alternatives (than homicide) to end an abusive and controlling relationship. Though laws have been introduced to limit gun ownership of those with domestic violence histories, men have still enjoyed the greatest reduction in rate of intimate partner homicide victimization. It is important to reiterate that previous intimate partner violence is the greatest risk factor for murder within a relationship. Efforts should be marshalled to prevent intimate partner violence. Thus, we will likely see a reduction in intimate partner homicide (especially among women).

References

1. Tjaden PG, Thoennes N. extent, nature, and consequences of intimate partner violence. NIJ Research Report/CDC. July 2000.
2. Vittes KA, Sorenson SB. Are temporary restraining orders more likely to be issued when applications mention firearms? Eval Rev. 2006;30(3):266–82.
3. Zeoli AM, Malinski R, Turchan B. Risks and targeted interventions: firearms in intimate partner violence. Epidemiol Rev. 2016;38(1):125–39. https://doi.org/10.1093/epirev/mxv007.
4. Vigdor ER, Mercy JA. Do laws restricting access to firearms by domestic violence offenders prevent intimate partner homicide? Eval Rev. 2006;30(3):313–46.
5. Nathan AJ. At the intersection of domestic violence and guns: the public interest exception and the Lautenberg amendment. Cornell L Rev. 1999;85:822.
6. Bachman R. A comparison of annual incidence rates and contextual characteristics of intimate-partner violence against women from the National Crime Victimization Survey (NCVS) and the National Violence Against Women Survey (NVAWS). Violence Against Women. 2000;6(8):839–67.
7. Wadman MC, Muelleman RL. Domestic violence homicides: ED use before victimization. Am J Emerg Med. 1999;17(7):689–91.
8. Campbell JC, Glass N, Sharps PW, Laughon K, Bloom T. Intimate partner homicide: review and implications of research and policy. Trauma Violence Abuse. 2007;8(3):246–69.
9. Beyer KM, Layde PM, Hamberger LK, Laud PW. Does neighborhood environment differentiate intimate partner femicides from other femicides? Violence Against Women. 2015;21(1):49–64.

10. Fox JA, Zawitz MW. Homicide trends in the United States. NCJ 204885. Washington, DC: U.S. Department of Justice, Bureau of Justice Statistics; 2004.
11. Wiebe DJ. Homicide and suicide risks associated with firearms in the home: a national case-control study. Ann Emerg Med. 2003;41(6):771–82.
12. Caman S, Kristiansson M, Granath S, Sturup J. Trends in rates and characteristics of intimate partner homicides between 1990 and 2013. J Crim Just. 2017;49:14–21.
13. Arbuckle J, Olson L, Howard M, Brillman J, Anctil C, Sklar D. Safe at home? Domestic violence and other homicides among women in New Mexico. Ann Emerg Med. 1996;27(2):210–5.
14. McFarlane J, Soeken K, Campbell J, Parker B, Reel S, Silva C. Severity of abuse to pregnant women and associated gun access of the perpetrator. Public Health Nurs. 1998;15(3):201–6.
15. Mercy JA, Saltzman LE. Fatal violence among spouses in the United States, 1976-85. Am J Public Health. 1989;79(5):595–9.

Intimate Partner Violence: Stalking

16

Theresa A. Bailey and Janice M. Beal

Stalking behavior is important to consider to insure a victim's safety once he or she escapes a violent intimate partner relationship. Stalking can diminish the feeling of autonomy and privacy both while in and after separating from an abusive relationship. Thus, it is important to know how this abusive behavior is often employed to ensure control and intimidation. Stalking can deter a victim from fleeing due to the feeling of helplessness and fear that it may create. In this chapter we will look at how some perpetrators of abuse use stalking as an emotional and physiological tactic to stoke fear in their victims. It is this fear of serious harm or even death that can often stifle victims and their advocates' efforts to separate from an abusive relationship.

Physical violence is not the only aspect of IPV. The abuse can take many diverse forms. Common manifestations of abusive behavior include imposing economic or financial restrictions, enforcing physical and emotional isolation, repeatedly invading the victim's privacy, supervising the victim's behavior, terminating support from family or friends, threatening violence toward the victim, threatening suicide, getting the victim addicted to drugs or alcohol, and physically or sexually assaulting the victim [1]. The perpetrator of abuse usually seeks to undermine his or her victim's autonomy. In keeping with this pattern of behavior, a perpetrator of abuse often deprives a victim of his or her consent or decision-making regarding matters involving his or her own body, life, work, and acquaintances [2, 3].

Intimate partner violence involves creating a pattern of interaction, with one's domestic partner or close relationship, in which the central theme is to create an atmosphere of dominance/control, create dependence, promote social isolation, and inhibit the victim's reality testing [4]. Physical violence is one of many methods employed to maintain power and control. It is this need for power and control that

T. A. Bailey (✉)
Bailey Psychiatric Associates, Houston, TX, USA
e-mail: office@baileypsych.com; theresa@baileypsych.com

J. M. Beal
Beal Counseling Associates, Houston, TX, USA

R. K. Bailey (ed.), *Intimate Partner Violence*,
https://doi.org/10.1007/978-3-030-55864-2_16

is the cornerstone of intimate partner violence perpetration. Intimate partner violence (IPV) differs from other forms of violent acts in that IPV tends to have a serial and repetitive nature. The National Violence Against Women Study found that 81% of women who were stalked by an intimate partner also experienced physical violence at the hands of that same partner [5]. This troubling result shows that just as there are tremendous physiological burdens when experiencing stalking, likely there is a concomitant physical abuse component occurring as well. Additionally, these acts of actual or threatened violence may often occur after separation or divorce. Sadly, IPV may only resolve upon the death of one or both partners. There is a body of evidence that indicates the pattern of increased violence (particularly lethal violence) that occurs once the abuser suspects an eminent attempt at or actual separation [5].

Attachment theory is a psychological model that may be useful in understanding the etiology of stalking behavior, as a dysfunctional development in early interpersonal relationships. It focuses on how people in relationships respond to hurt or threat (such as a breakup) within a relationship. Some understanding can be gleaned from attachment theory as to why an individual may illogically use stalking after and during the dissolution of a relationship [5]. Often stalking is done to spite the opposition from the other partner. Opposition can be verbal or legal expressions (such as orders of protection or divorce). Some have looked to attachment theory to explain this maladaptive behavior as the stalker's attempt to gain proximity to the victim and thus somehow strengthen his/her chances to retain the relationship. Therefore, some predictors of perpetrating stalking behaviors have been identified in abusers' personal history. One of these is a history of early attachment disruptions in childhood, as well as perceived losses or separation in the course of adult intimate relationships [6]. So when faced with a possible loss or separation, an intimate partner/stalker may attempt to isolate his or her partner to maintain control and diminish his or her autonomy, i.e., make it increasingly difficult to separate.

Leaving, moving on, separation, and divorce – these are all words that seem to set in motion a dangerous series of events for victims of IPV. It is in this transition that stalking becomes more prevalent. There is a very troubling correlation between stalking behavior and subsequent physical violence and murder. Indeed, stalking may be a noteworthy precursor to murder. More than 75% of murdered women were stalked [7]. Additionally, two-thirds of women who were physically assaulted, by either a partner or former partner, were within a year either murdered or a victim of attempted murder [7]. This points out that even though a victim may have separated from an abusive partner, he or she is not yet safe. Separation is a dangerous transitional period for a victim of IPV [7].

IPV can be physical as well as psychological. A particular type of psychological IPV is stalking. The following statistic makes the relationship between stalking and violence disturbingly clear. Eighty percent (80%) of reported stalking of intimate partners had concomitant physical violence. Furthermore, 76 percent (76%) of all women who were killed by their intimate partner were also stalked by that partner [8].

The 2010 National Intimate Partner and Sexual Violence Survey describes stalking as unwanted behavior performed by a perpetrator that causes fear or safety concerns for a victim [4]. In the survey, stalking tactics measured were:

- Unwanted phone calls, voice or text messages, hang-ups
- Unwanted emails, instant messages, messages through social media
- Unwanted cards, letters, flowers, or presents
- Watching or following from a distance, spying with a listening device, camera, or global positioning system (GPS)
- Approaching or showing up in places such as the victim's home, workplace, or school when it was unwanted
- Leaving strange or potentially threatening items for the victim to find
- Sneaking into a victim's home or car and doing things to scare the victim or let the victim know the perpetrator had been there [4]

Having an understanding of stalking tactics used by perpetrators, victim advocates will have facts to be alerted of possible impending violence. Likewise, we can highlight and point out some disturbing statistics. Per the 2010 survey, about one in six women experienced stalking in their lifetime [4]. Importantly, women were more likely than men to report being "very fearful" that she or someone close to her would be harmed or even killed [4]. Although much less likely than women, men reported being stalked as well. Per the 2015 updated survey, approximately 1 in 19 men reported that they had been victimized by means of stalking during their lifetime [9]. This equates to about 5.9 million men (survey of men in the United States). Likewise, men who were stalked also reported being "very fearful" that he or someone close to him would be harmed or even killed [9]. This highlights that the stalker's messages of fear, even from afar, resonate with each victim regardless of gender.

When an intimate partner is stalking his or her victim, a number of stalking tactics are used. The most universal of these tactics is sending unwanted phone calls, voice or text messages, or hang-ups. Thus, it makes it exceedingly important to understand that abuse can take many diverse forms. Common manifestations of that behavior include imposing economic or financial restrictions, enforcing physical and emotional isolation, repeatedly invading the victim's privacy, supervising the victim's behavior, terminating support from family or friends, threatening violence toward the victim, threatening suicide, getting the victim addicted to drugs or alcohol, and physically or sexually assaulting the victim [1].

Over half of female stalking victims reported that stalking first occurred before the age of 25. This accounts for about 10.4 million victims [9]. Dating violence and IPV happen among adolescents and young adults at high rates. According to the 2015 National Intimate Partner and Sexual Violence Survey, over half of women and 41% of males who were surveyed reported being stalked before the age of 25 years old [9]. The use of surveillance technology and electronic communication as a method of stalking is referred to as cyberstalking. Cyberstalking is often used to bully and shame victims in this age population. Thus teenagers and young adults, particularly females, are an important group to glean some understanding on the dynamics of IPV, stalking, and technology.

Cyberstalking can be defined as the use of electronic-based communication to enact behaviors such as repeated threats or harassment intended to make the victim afraid or concerned for his or her safety [4]. Some examples of cyberstalking are monitoring email or social media communication either directly on the victim's computer or through covert programs; sending email that threatens, insults, or harasses; using the victim's email identity to send false messages to others or to purchase goods and services; and using the Internet to seek and compile a victim's personal information for use in harassment [4]. Additionally, spyware can be installed on a victim's computer. Spyware can potentially record every key typed, including all passwords, PIN numbers, websites, and email. If possible, a victim of abuse may need to use a public computer such as those available in a library, to avoid such cyber-intrusions.

Monitoring the misuse of technology is problematic as society and all its components continue to become increasingly more digital. Many important transactions such as banking, travel, education, and social interactions occur online. Spyware that may allow a perpetrator of abuse/IPV to be privy to this information could potentially thwart any attempt by the victim to gain privacy or escape. For example, it was reported in an article that a victim of cyberstalking by her ex-husband was boldly shown the evidence he obtained, "he presented the computer information to prove that he could violate her sense of security whenever and wherever he wanted, even after he moved out of the region" [10]. Statements like these create a bleak outlook for victims of cyberstalking. It almost elevates the perpetrator of abuse to an omnipresent omnipotent entity. Naturally, this can be very disheartening for someone who is considering leaving an abuser.

By embracing technology, stalkers can employ innovative and disturbing ways to harass their victims, creating a scenario where abusers can harass victims by proxy. For example, in 1999, Gary Dellapenta harassed his ex-girlfriend by proxy. He began to impersonate his girlfriend online. He would enter chat rooms and dating websites. Posing as his ex-girlfriend, he would tell of elaborate and explicit rape fantasies. In addition to encouraging strangers to help her fulfill her rape fantasy, Dellapenta posted his ex-girlfriend's name and home address. Six men ultimately were enticed by what appeared to be open advances. These men showed up at Dellapenta's ex-girlfriend's residence presumably to participate in the rape fantasy. This created a terrifying circumstance for the victim. Fortunately, Dellapenta was ultimately arrested [11]. However, more sophisticated stalkers could use methods such as anonymous remailers and make it practically impossible to be detected and subsequently prosecuted [12].

The use of technology to instill fear and to gain some sense of proximity to their victims is a significant factor to consider in the study of intimate partner violence and stalking, particularly as we examine younger victims. There are good uses of technology; victims may use online resources to help successfully escape their controlling and ever vigilant abusers. However more often than not, technology has made it easier for abusers to spy on their victims, especially if they no longer cohabitate. Understanding this dichotomy is important to better aid victims. Indeed, stalking and harassment may seem inescapable for some. Thus, it becomes important to know how perpetrators of abuse can use technology to control, intimidate, and keep tabs on their victims. Furthermore, teenagers are a high-risk group for IPV and have a great online presence as well. Adolescents are often inundated with information from their peers that influences their thought on relationships, social norms, and partner violence.

Technology can often be a double-edged sword regarding IPV. Every new technological service offers an opportunity for a victim to inconspicuously gather information and possibly escape abuse. Sadly, this same technology can be utilized maliciously by perpetrators of IPV with disastrous consequences for their victims. For example, a New England woman had mustered the courage to leave her abusive husband. She had been diligent in gathering information and resources to flee. She had found a new home for herself and her two children. With all her plans carefully in place, she sent an email to a friend asking for help during her move. She was cautious enough to delete this communication. However, the email still lingered in her "deleted mail" folder. Unfortunately, her husband found the email. Upon learning of her plans to escape, he became enraged and killed her [4].

As society has become more technology centered, so too has stalking in the context of intimate partner abuse. Many perpetrators of IPV are turning to technology to exact their influence. Sadly, this flagrant disregard for personal boundaries lends itself well to stalking. This disregard for the privacy of an intimate partner or former intimate partner has evolved at the same rapidity as technology. Cyberstalking, the use of technology such as GPS, spyware computer programs, cell phone monitoring chips, and tiny surveillance cameras, can often be used by perpetrators to track the locations, activities, and communications of their victims. Sadly, detailed statistics of cyberstalking are unavailable. The issue is likely underreported due to the difficulty in identifying and/or detecting it. Thus, new considerations of the law, public policy, and online service provider must be made when addressing this newer component of IPV. Technology has become ever more sophisticated. Innovations intended to enhance communication and safety such as the Internet, global positioning systems, and surveillance equipment are now potential implements that can be used to stalk, intimidate, and control. Now domestic violence victim advocates must be also savvy to the ways technology can ensnare victims. This must be taken into consideration for safety planning [4].

The act of stalking itself only became criminalized in 1990 [4]. California was the first state to pass an anti-stalking law in 1990. Interestingly enough, the law was established in response to the murder of actress Rebecca Schaeffer and five other Orange County women who were stalked and murdered by former intimate partners [4]. Three years later, all 50 states had laws that prohibited stalking [13]. This was after the issue gained media attention in the late 1980s and 1990s [14]. Before the implementation of such laws, law enforcement could do little to insure safety or privacy of stalking victims [15]. This surge of stalking in public awareness has led some to refer to stalking as "the crime of the 1990s" [16].

The criminal justice system is without an effective tool to combat cyberstalking. As technology continues to rapidly become more and more sophisticated, perpetrators may find it easier to escape detection, apprehension, and prosecution. Here are some figures that show the established link between cyberstalking/stalking and IPV. Twenty-six percent (26%) of all stalking victims reported that they were stalked by technological means [8]. The American criminal justice system has made tremendous strides in the recognition and prosecution of intimate partner violence. However, there is still much to be done, particularly in how we should now interpret existing laws regarding free speech, privacy, age of consent, and age of criminal responsibility, in arenas of both criminal law and tort laws – especially when technology is utilized to commit assault through cyberstalking and bullying.

Sadly, teenagers and young adults under 25 years old are becoming a large pool of IPV victims, particularly cyberstalking and bullying. The literature suggests that historically law enforcement has not adequately responded to cyberstalking [8], particularly when no physical violence has occurred. In the United States, nearly all teenagers use technology (cell phone, computers). Also, technology is being used socially as a platform in expressing sexual identity and intimate emotions [8]. This ubiquitous use of technology can influence a teenager's development, particularly at the stage of development when teenagers are transitioning from relying on their parents for information and looking more to peers to inform their behavior. In the process of growing into adults, navigating society, understanding relationships, and developing an identity, teenagers differentiate themselves from their parents. In doing so the influence of their peers becomes magnified and exalted. Thus, it becomes exceedingly important to know that behavior (even online) may have a profound influence on teenagers and young adults. Indeed, even the Supreme Court of the United States has recognized that teenagers often demonstrate a "lack of maturity," greater susceptibility to peer pressure, and more fluid characters [17]. This time of self-discovery and transition may impart lasting views on relationships. Indeed, dating during teenage years is important in learning skills such as communication, empathy, and compromise. Many in mid/late adolescence report spending more time with their romantic partner than with friends or family [18]. Moreover, teenagers often look to peers to get information on interpersonal relationships. They gauge what is appropriate based largely on the reactions of their friends. Coupled with this time of tremendous personal growth is the potential for great risk. Adolescents who are dating are at the greatest risk for IPV for any age group [18]. Approximately one third of adolescent girls are victims of physical, emotional, or verbal abuse from a dating partner [18].

Most teenagers use online services and programs/apps without adult supervision [8]. This lack of supervision may lead to unhealthy/unsafe online behavior. Thus many unkind and frankly inappropriate conversations, pictures, and videos that would not be spoken or done face to face are normalized in an unsupervised online world. This may lead to a more permissive/accepting attitude toward cyberstalking and other menacing online behavior. Thus, young people's expectation of privacy may be diminished. This can be coupled with a more cavalier behavior often adopted by those while communicating online. This can set up a high-risk environment for abusive behavior. Thus, some may be reasonably hesitant to scrutinize, sanction, or criminalize "normal teenage behavior." Appropriately, there is concern about the possibility of the next generation normalizing unhealthy relationship behavior while espousing technology. As stated earlier, technology can be a tool to exert control and intimidate.

The criminal justice system may be at the cusp of a potential crisis, as more and more aggressive/inappropriate online engagements go unchecked. The authorities – lawmakers, law enforcement, and parents – do not appear to grasp the potential harm, gravity of violence, and aggressive behavior that occur among adolescent and young adult relationships, particularly in the cyberworld. Much is dismissed as "normal behavior." An initial starting point to help remedy the problem would be to create awareness. Hopefully, increased awareness will ensure that law enforcement and parents recognize the seriousness of online behavior (threats, stalking, and humiliation) and do away with flippant and dismissive attitudes regarding this matter. Thankfully, over the past 30 years, society as a whole has become more aware of the existence of domestic violence. Indeed, this increased awareness of domestic violence has led to criminalization of domestic violence at the state and federal levels. Hopefully, increased awareness will aid in criminalizing the assaultive engagements that occur in cyberworld.

Technology has helped people to connect with one another. Communication between individuals is now instantaneous. Technology can play a role in allowing a victim of IPV to discreetly get support as well as information to flee. However, technology can also aid the controlling and power-hungry perpetrators. Technology has made surveillance of others easier than ever. Most components of daily life such as shopping, consumption of news, communication, job searching, banking, and travel booking all occur online. This information is often used by perpetrators of abuse to control and isolate their victims. Additionally, teenagers are at the forefront of technology use. They are very likely to be influenced by their peers. Regrettably, many bad maladaptive habits regarding control, power, respect, communication, and empathy develop during adolescent years. Inappropriate engagements may be glorified by a teenager's online community and set the stage for creating the next generation of either abusers or victims. Teenagers experience high levels of IPV. Their online activity is often unsupervised and may be a platform for abuse and the normalization of abuse.

References

1. King-Ries A. Teens, technology, and cyberstalking: the domestic violence wave of the future. Tex J Women L. 2010;20:131.
2. Kurt JL. Stalking as a variant of domestic violence. J Am Acad Psychiatry Law Online. 1995;23(2):219–30.
3. Mullen PE, Pathe M, Purcell R, Stuart GW. A study of stalkers. Am J Psychiatry. 1999;156:1244–9.
4. Black M, Basile K, Breiding M, Smith S, Walters M, Merrick M, Chen J, Stevens M. National intimate partner and sexual violence survey: 2010 summary report.
5. Mechanic MB, Weaver TL, Resick PA. Intimate partner violence and stalking behavior: exploration of patterns and correlates in a sample of acutely battered women. Violence Vict. 2000;15(1):55–72.

6. Douglas KS, Dutton DG. Assessing the link between stalking and domestic violence. Aggress Violent Behav. 2001;6(6):519–46.
7. Mechanic MB, Uhlmansiek MH, Weaver TL, Resick PA. The impact of severe stalking experienced by acutely battered women: an examination of violence, psychological symptoms and strategic responding. Violence Vict. 2000;15(4):443.
8. Sheridan L, Davies GM. Stalking: the elusive crime. Legal Criminal Psychol. 2001;6(2):133–47.
9. Smith SG, Zhang X, Basile KC, Merrick MT, Wang J, Kresnow MJ, Chen J. The national intimate partner and sexual violence survey: 2015 data brief–updated release.
10. Meloy JR. Stalking (obsessional following): a review of some preliminary studies. Aggress Violent Behav. 1996;1(2):147–62.
11. Grodzinsky FS, Tavani HT. Some ethical reflections on cyberstalking. ACM SIGCAS Comp Soc. 2002;32(1):22–32.
12. Spitzberg BH, Hoobler G. Cyberstalking and the technologies of interpersonal terrorism. New Media Soc. 2002;4(1):71–92.
13. Southworth C, Finn J, Dawson S, Fraser C, Tucker S. Intimate partner violence, technology, and stalking. Violence Against Women. 2007;13(8):842–56.
14. Bjerregaard B. An empirical study of stalking victimization. Violence Vict. 2000;15(4):389.
15. Emerson RM, Ferris KO, Gardner CB. On being stalked. Soc Probl. 1998;45(3):289–314.
16. Gilligan MJ. Stalking the stalker: developing new laws to thwart those who terrorize others. Ga L Rev. 1992;27:285.
17. Lerner CS. Sentenced to confusion: Miller v. Alabama and the coming wave of Eighth Amendment Cases. Geo Mason L Rev. 2012;20:25.
18. Glass N, Fredland N, Campbell J, Yonas M, Sharps P, Kub J. Adolescent dating violence: prevalence, risk factors, health outcomes, and implications for clinical practice. J Obstet Gynecol Neonatal Nurs. 2003;32(2):227–38.

17 Substance Abuse and Intimate Partner Violence

Dashiel J. Geyen and Rahn Kennedy Bailey

Introduction

Depressants, stimulants, hallucinogens, opioids, inhalants, cannabis, and alcohol are all agents that when consumed by humans can influence their behaviors. A person's behavior may be persuaded by these psychoactive substances often resulting in changes and distortions in their sensations, perceptions, and reality. Not only do these chemicals have a direct effect on a person's behavior; they can also impact the lives of other people.

It seems as though substance use has become an integral part of society. For certain drugs, such as cannabis, there appears to be a greater leniency for it and more acceptance of its use. For example, in North America, there are 33 states as well as the District of Colombia which have passed regulations broadly legalizing the use of Cannabis for medical and/or recreational purposes [1].

Cannabidiol oil, a marijuana derivative, has become a very popular product. Its sale is grossing hundreds of thousands of dollars in many states in America mostly for reported medicinal reasons. This drug is being widely manufactured and distributed throughout the country. The caveat is that cannabidiol oil is not regulated by the US Food and Drug Administration. Consequently, the product is subject to variation in content and quality.

Although there is what appears to be a growing trend in the United States to tolerate substance use, there are also those who are very concerned as to the undesirable influence that substance use may have on many American citizens. Substance

D. J. Geyen (✉)
Prairie View A & M University, Prairie View, TX, USA
e-mail: rahnkbaileymd@comcast.net

R. K. Bailey
Department of Psychiatry, Charles R. Drew University of Medicine and Science, Los Angeles, CA, USA

R. K. Bailey (ed.), *Intimate Partner Violence*,
https://doi.org/10.1007/978-3-030-55864-2_17

use unfortunately is often associated with occurrence of tragic events throughout the populace.

For example, according to the Centers for Disease Control, everyday 29 people in the United States die in motor vehicle crashes that involve an alcohol-inebriated driver. That is one death every 50 minutes [2].

In addition, substance use is often connected to incidents of child abuse and neglect.

It was reported that in the Corpus Christi Caller-Times in July 2018, a Corpus Christi, Texas mother sold her son for $2500.00 to resolve a drug money debt [3].

Substance use effects employment among able-bodied individuals. Jackie Calmes a writer for the New York Times reported that across the nation, employers are wanting to hire workers. However, the applicants are unable to pass the initial drug test. The companies who are hiring workers want to avoid the risk of liability. Furthermore, businesses like trucking companies are required by federal law to drug test their employees for safety reasons [4].

Substance use is often notoriously connected with violent behaviors. The consumption of alcohol and illicit drugs are more likely to promote aggressive behaviors among its users. Research has suggested that there are certain drugs which are intimately associated with aggression among its users.

In one study, investigators wanted to know if methamphetamine use increases violent behaviors. Moreover, according to the National Institute on Drug Abuse, methamphetamines are a manufactured powerful highly addicted stimulus that affects the central nervous system. The researchers found that there were observable changes in behaviors, whereas subjects were becoming aggressive during periods of methamphetamine use. Violent behavior was 6.2 times more likely to occur when subjects were using methamphetamines relative to when they were not using the drug [5].

In can be easily noted how many different ways in which substance use can impose stress and hardship on an individual. One way involves the nature of a relationship between two people who are intimately connected. Therefore, this paper will examine the concept of intimate partner violence and substance abuse. More specifically, it will distinguish between substance use and substance abuse. The essay will also explore and discuss some central behavioral characteristics of the perpetrator and the victim as it relates to substance use with intimate partners. Finally, it will offer two clinical case study vignettes used to illustrate and profile characteristics of the perpetrator/substance use. Additionally, the study includes the victim and substance use, all of which centers around intimate partner violence.

Intimate Partner Violence

For the purpose of this essay, intimate partner violence (IPV) may be conceptualized as physically aggressive type behaviors transpiring between two people in a close liaison. The term "intimate partner" denotes a current or former spouse, monogamous relationship, or dating relationship where there is a physical attraction as well as an emotional connection [6].

According to the Centers for Disease Control and Prevention, intimate partner violence describes physical, sexual, or psychological harm by a current or former partner or spouse. This type of violence can occur among heterosexual or same-sex couples, and it does not require sexual intimacy.

More specifically intimate partner violence may be categorized into four types: physical violence occurs when one individual in the relationship intentionally hurts or attempts to hurt their partner by kicking, hitting, or using any type of physical force. The second type is sexual violence. It is when one person forces or attempts to force their partner to take part in a sex act or sexual touching. Sexual violence is also nonphysical sexual contact when their partner does not or cannot give consent. Such is the case with sexting on cellular phones [6].

The third form of intimate partner violence is called stalking. Stalking is a pattern of continuous unwanted attention and contact by a partner that causes fear, apprehension, or a problem for one's own safety as well as the well-being of someone close to or related to the victim. The fourth category is called psychological aggression. This is the use of verbal or nonverbal communication with the intent to harm the victim mentally or emotionally in an effort to exert control of their behavior [6].

These different types of intimate partner violence can occur simultaneously. It causes the victim great emotional discomfort, physical pain, and mental distress. The Centers for Disease Control and Prevention indicates victims of intimate partner violence are at a much greater risk for engaging in behaviors like smoking, illicit drug abuse, and alcohol binge drinking [6].

Substance Use Disorder

Substance use disorder is a combination of cognitive, behavioral, emotional, and physiological activities that continues to interfere and impacts an individual's normal way of adaptive functioning. According to the *Diagnostic and Statistical Manual of Mental Disorder – Fifth Edition*, one of the most salient issues of substance use disorder occurs in brain chemistry [7]. Moreover, nearly all of the addictive type drugs either directly or indirectly focus on the brain's reward system by flooding the circuit with dopamine.

The reward system is comprised of the main dopamine pathways of the brain that include the mesolimbic pathways, the ventral tegmental area (VTA), and the nucleus accumbens [8].

Dopamine is a neurotransmitter that has the responsibility of regulating movement, emotion, cognition, motivation, and the reinforcement of rewarding behaviors. Under normal circumstances, the reward system complements natural behaviors. However, overstimulating the system with drug use creates the effects that reinforce repeated drug use behaviors [8]. These chemical changes in the brain can continue even after a person has undergone drug detoxification.

Individuals who have substance abuse disorders may show unsubstantiated lability of mood even when the situation does not warrant such a change in emotions. They may present with what is considered observable symptoms of unstable affect. Furthermore, people with substance use disorder may exhibit obsessive thoughts patterns centered around the next time they are able to use drugs. Many times, their behaviors are linked to their obsessive thought. Behaviors are generally motivated by the desire to use the substance again. These compulsive kinds of behaviors can interfere with a person's ability attend to family, work, school, etc.

Substance Abuse

In 2019, the World Health Organization defined substance abuse as the harmful or hazardous use of psychoactive substances, including alcohol and illicit drugs. Psychoactive substance use can lead to a dependence syndrome, which involves a cluster of behavioral, cognitive, and physiological phenomena that develop after repeated substance use [9].

Substance abuse is self-destructive, and it generally includes a dominating desire to continue to take the alcohol or illicit drug despite the harmful effects and consequences. A person who abuses alcohol or illicit drugs exhibit difficulties controlling its use; moreover the individual will place a higher priority on drug use than other activities and obligations. The person is subject to increased tolerance of the substance and sometimes may go into a physical withdrawal state. It is particularly so when they no longer use alcohol or illicit drugs.

This behavior is seen, whereas an individual will be facing legal problems as a result of their abusing alcohol or illicit drugs. The person could face criminal charges for vehicular manslaughter after being involved in an automobile accident while under the influence of alcohol. In addition, the individual made a gross driving error while maneuvering their car causing a major collision of other vehicles. This resulted in the driver and the passenger in the other car being killed, and, more often, this would not have been the first time a person has had encounters with the legal systems as a result of alcohol abuse.

In a related incident, stories are often reported of the person who is a drug abuser and becomes violent toward others. There were cases where innocent people were shot and wounded or even became victims of assault. Alcohol and illicit drugs are always a part of the crime scene.

Drugs and Alcohol and the Victim

The individual who sustains the painful and powerful outcomes of an abusive relationship is called the victim. Generally, the victim is a female in a heterosexual relationship. According to a US Surgeon General's report in 2003, the National Violence Against Women Survey, one of four women in the United States has been physically assaulted or raped by an intimate partner [10].

The report went on to suggest that every year, an estimated four million women are physically abused by their spouses and live-in partners. Among those women who are subjected to physical assault and rape, one in three is injured and requires medical treatment [10].

Assault is a traumatic experience for many women. It therefore causes a great deal of cognitive and emotional distress for the female victim. Consequently, these women will often resort to substance use and substance abuse. Much of the research has indicated that the anger, fear, and humiliation that a woman experiences in an abusive relationship may provoke drug use [12]. The use of alcohol and illicit drugs can alter their state of consciousness and thereby ease the physical and emotional pain they experience.

A victim may be persuasively coerced into using alcohol and illicit drugs as a manipulation tactic employed by the perpetrator that is used in an intimate partner violent relationship. The victim is led to believe that engaging in such activity with the perpetrator will strengthen the bond of their relationship. It is essential to understand the addictive nature of alcohol and illicit drugs and the impact they have on human behavior. Over a period of time with continued use, it could lead to a "double" dependency. That is, the victim not only becomes dependent on the substances used but on the dysfunctional connection with the perpetrator as well.

There are often other integral pieces of human behavior which are connected to domestic violence along with continued substance use. Personal characteristics such as having low self-esteem, poor self-confidence, and a lack of impulse control can be interrelated to this type of situation. Circumstantial influences such as money, community, culture, and family can be contributors to female victims of substance abuse and intimate partner violence.

Madison has dealt with symptoms of depression, poor self-esteem, and a lack of self-confidence since middle school. She and her sister have been victims of neglect and abused during her early school years. Madison's immediate family life was chaotic and unstable. Her father had been in federal penitentiary for illegally transporting people into the United States. Consequently, he had difficulty getting housing and finding gainful employment for his family. Madison's father was often away from home and would remain away for several days at a time.

Madison's mother had chronic health problems. She too was away from home, in and out of jail for soliciting and selling illicit drugs. Madison's mother claimed she was forced to sell drugs to get money to support the family. Madison was placed in foster care with a distant relative.

As an adolescent, Madison had begun to experiment with drugs and alcohol. Although she would often isolate herself from others, she became involved with a group of peers who were stagnate in their development. At the age of 17, she met Conrad.

Conrad was 24 years old and a truck driver. They started out as sexual partners; however, their relationship began to grow more and more intimate. At age 18 Madison got pregnant with Conrad's child. Consequently, Madison left her foster care home and moved into an apartment with Conrad. After 3 months Madison miscarried the pregnancy.

Madison became depressed as a result of all the events which had occurred in her life. She and Conrad would use drugs and alcohol recreationally. However, Madison said that she was only using drugs and alcohol to numb her depressed feelings.

For about 2 or 3 days prior to his leaving to make a delivery out of town driving the truck, Conrad would not use any drugs or alcohol. He said this would give him time to "clean it out." Conrad would sometimes stay away from Madison for several weeks at a time. He would drive the truck from one city to another before returning home. While he was away, Madison would not interact much with friends or family. She would work part-time or short-term jobs. Conrad did not want her to work outside of the house. Instead he wanted her to have children.

Conrad was now becoming more controlling of Madison. Before he would depart for one of his extended trips, Conrad would only leave Madison with a designated amount of money to live on. He maintains control of their bank account, and she would have to get permission from him to gain access to it. He would note the mileage on their car before he left and would question her tremendously if it seemed to him that she had used the car too much.

Madison and Conrad would frequently engage in sexual intercourse prior to his leaving on a road trip. He forbade her to use any kinds of birth control or contraceptives. It was Conrad's intention to impregnate Madison. This was Conrad's assurance that Madison would not become intimate with another man, when he was away from home.

Repeatedly, upon his initial return home after being away for an extended period, Conrad would spend time using alcohol and illicit drugs. He wanted Madison to join him. To avoid Conrad's anger outbursts and his threats to harm her, Madison would participate in drug and alcohol use with him. Madison was very unhappy with her current lifestyle.

Drugs and Alcohol and the Perpetrator

The person who incites violent behaviors in an intimate partner violent relationship is referred to as the perpetrator. There is no single or definitive profile of a perpetrator; however, the perpetrator typically is a male. He can be a member of any race or ethnic group. The perpetrator may come from any socioeconomic strata, religious group, or educational assemblage. However, one factor that is believed to contribute to aggressive behavior is the use of alcohol and drugs.

Alcohol and drugs are chemicals that can interfere with normal flow of neural activity within the brain. These chemicals subject to change a person's perception and reactions. Under the influence of alcohol or illicit drugs, a perpetrator can become less inhibited and more likely to portray poor judgment, irrational behaviors, and weak impulse control. It is important to note however, that Bancroft reported that not all substance users are abusive partners nor are all abusive partners substance users in intimate partner relationships [13].

Research has suggested there is a connection between substance use and intimate partner violence perpetration. Alcohol and drug use – particularly cocaine and methamphetamines – are thought to be constant risk factors for intimate partner violence perpetuation [14]. Cocaine and methamphetamines tend to overstimulate the nervous system. The drugs tend to increase the amount of dopamine in the brain. Although the result is usually a pleasurable feeling, the drugs could cause an individual to become impulsive, anxious, aggressive, and exhibiting a sense of power and control [8]. Its use has also been linked to violent behaviors.

The perpetrator's drug or alcohol use may be coupled with other behavioral characteristics. They may suffer from low self-esteem and a poor self-concept. Perpetrators tend to be controlling and manipulative. These individuals have an extreme need to maintain power and domination over their partners. Males who have been identified with personality disorders such as narcissistic, histrionic, borderline, and antisocial tend to be more characteristic of an intimate partner violent perpetrator.

Leviticus is a 30-year-old male. He is from a midsized city in the southern region of the United States. Leviticus grew up in what may be described as a marginally dysfunctional family environment. There had been reported cases of child neglect of him and his siblings; however, subsequent reports found no evidence. There have also been illegal allegations made toward members of his family for theft and illicit drug use.

Leviticus participated in high school sports and from all indications was a talented athlete. His coaches said that Leviticus had the potential to compete at the college level, if he would have more disciplined and dedicated.

Nevertheless, Leviticus completed high school and went on to complete a heating, ventilation, and air-conditioning certification in a local community college. He was a recreational drug user. He liked to smoke marijuana and drink alcohol regularly. He would frequently use cocaine. Leviticus never perceived his drug and alcohol use as a problem. He knew that once under the influence of these substances, it changes his thinking and behavior. However, he did not seek any professional help. Leviticus was known to harbor a great deal of self-doubt in his own abilities. He tends to give up easily if he perceives that a task was too difficult. In many respects, he could be controlling and was known to manipulate his friends into getting things he wanted.

One summer day afternoon, while attending a holiday barbeque at his relative's home, Leviticus met Jeanine. Jeanine was a college student, and she worked part-time at a local firm. They became more acquainted and over time formulated a relationship. Jeanine was outgoing and had a warm and friendly disposition. She had attractive physical characteristics and enjoyed social interactions, all of the characteristics that Leviticus found appealing.

On the other hand, Jeanine liked the attention that Leviticus gave to her. He would invite her on dates. They would attend movies, concerts, and theatrical plays together. He was also good with helping with things like car repairs and other odd jobs.

In the midst of their romance, the couple decided to move in together. Their relationship continued, and for a while, things appeared to be going well. Jeanine was aware of Leviticus's drug and alcohol use. She would on occasions take part in the drug and alcohol use with him.

Jeanine soon became concern about the impact that their drug use was having on their lifestyle as well as their relationship. Leviticus was developing a tolerance for alcohol and drugs. Consequently, he was using more and more alcohol as well as drugs. It was costing the couple increasing amounts of money.

When Leviticus had been using drugs and alcohol, his behavior would change. Jeanine said that Leviticus would become belligerent and hostile if things didn't go his way. He was becoming increasingly controlling and manipulative toward Jeanine. She had even stopped using alcohol and drugs. Leviticus was very critical of Jeanine's mode of dress, her hairstyle, and body shape. These behaviors were even more pronounced after he had been drinking alcohol and using drugs.

Conclusion

Intimate partner violence and substance use are a public health concern. This deadly combination creates an estimated cost well into the millions of dollars across the nation. It impacts and destroys the lives of countless numbers of individuals, several of which often result in death.

This essay begins with addressing the prevalence of substance use throughout society. It then continued with a discussion and conceptualization of intimate partner violence. In addition, the paper noted that substance use disorder is a combination of cognitive, behavioral, emotional, and physiological activities that continue to interfere and impact an individual's normal manner of adaptive functioning. Substance abuse is defined as a harmful or hazardous use of psychoactive substances, including alcohol and illicit drugs.

Information was presented on the existence of illicit drugs, alcohol, and their connections to the victim, the perpetrator, and the matter of intimate partner violence. Authentic case study vignettes were presented. They offered clinical illustrations of the dynamics occurring between couples in an intimate partner violent relationship.

References

1. Pacula RL, Smart R. Medical marijuana and marijuana legalization. Annu Rev Clin Psychol. 2017;13:397–419. https://doi.org/10.1146/annurev-clinpsy-032816-045128.
2. Impaired Driving: Get the Facts;. Motor Vehicle Safety; CDC Injury Center. https://www.cdc.gov/motorvehiclesafety/impaired_driving/impaired-drv_factsheet.html
3. Corpus Christi mother sold her son for $2,500.00 to clear a drug money debt. Monica Lopez; Corpus Christi Caller Times, July 2018.
4. Hiring hurdle: finding workers who can pass a drug test. Jackie Calmes; New York Times, May 2016.
5. McKetin R, Lubman DI, Najman JM, Dawe S, Butterworth P, Baker AL. Does methamphetamine use increase violent behavior? Evidence from a prospective longitudinal study. Addiction. 2014;109(5):798–806. https://doi.org/10.1111/add.12474.
6. Preventing Intimate Partner Violence. https://www.cdc.gov/violenceprevention/intimatepartnerviolence/fastfact.html

7. American Psychiatric Association. Diagnostic and statistical manual of mental disorders. 5th ed. Washington, DC; 2013.
8. Wise RP. Drug activation of brain reward pathways. Drug Alcohol Depend. 1998;51(1–2):13–22.
9. World Health Organization Health Topics: Substance Abuse https://www.who.int/topics/substance_abuse/en/
10. Rivera EA, Phillips H, Warshaw C, Lyon E, Bland PJ, Kaewken O. An applied research paper on the relationship between intimate partner violence and substance use. National Center on Domestic Violence, Trauma & Mental Health: Chicago, IL; 2015.
11. The full report on the prevalence incidence and consequences of violence against women. Findings from the National Violence Against Women Survey. https://www.ncjrs.gov/pdffiles1/nij/183781.pdf
12. Gilbert L, El-Bassel N, Schilling RF, Friedman E. Childhood abuse as a risk for partner abuse among women in Methadone Maintenance. Am J Drug Alcohol Abuse. 1997;23(4):581–95.
13. Bancroft L. Why does he do that? Inside the minds of angry and controlling men. New York: The Berkley Publishing Group; a division of Penguin Group; 2002.
14. Brecht ML, Herbeck DM. Methamphetamine use and violent behavior: user perception and predictors. J Drug Issues. 2013;43(4):468–82. https://doi.org/10.1177/0022042613491098.

18 Intimate Partner Violence During SARS-CoV-2 (COVID-19) Pandemic

Mallory Williams and Rahn Kennedy Bailey

Perhaps, there has been no greater impact on the context in which victims experience violence than that of the SARS-CoV-2 (COVID-19) pandemic. Mandated social policies that confine individuals to their domicile with their abuser greatly increase the opportunity for injury to victims. Estimates from the United Nations Population Fund suggest that 90 days of quarantine will result in a 20% global rise in IPV which is equivalent to 15 million new cases [1]. Key factors that drive these data are social isolation, stress, substance abuse, economic anxiety, and lack of accessible public resources for intervention.

Social Isolation

Social isolation is defined as a state of being cut off from normal social networks. This can be the result of a loss of mobility, unemployment, or health-related issues. COVID-19 can lead to all of the causes of social isolation. Social isolation is one of the most common maneuvers performed on victims by their abusers. Once confined to a known location with an abuser, the risks of IPV can be exceedingly high [2, 3]. Furthermore, the ability for outside influences to intervene is low. In essence, COVID-19 or any other natural disaster that confines individuals with their abusers

M. Williams (✉)
Howard University Hospital, Washington, DC, USA

Howard University College of Medicine, Washington, DC, USA

Howard University National Center of Excellence for Trauma & Violence Prevention, Washington, DC, USA
e-mail: mallwilliams@huhosp.org

R. K. Bailey
Department of Psychiatry, Charles R. Drew University of Medicine and Science, Los Angeles, CA, USA

R. K. Bailey (ed.), *Intimate Partner Violence*,
https://doi.org/10.1007/978-3-030-55864-2_18

creates the preferred scenario for the abuser. Victims become susceptible to both physical and emotional abuse such as the practice of *gaslighting*. The term gaslighting originates from a 1938 stage play entitled *Gas Light*. The abuser seeks to exert power and control over the victim by having them doubt their thoughts and feelings and thereby defer to their abuser. This creates a dependence that only more complicates the victim's ability to break free of the cycle of abuse. This of course is greatly facilitated by the lack of external encouraging or reassuring influences. James et al. (2004) in a social network study found that many of the women experienced physical and emotional aspects of isolation [4]. Furthermore, in each of these cases, this isolation was forced on these women [4]. Women with higher levels of social support are less likely to be victims of IPV, and this holds true across levels of neighborhood deprivation [5]. COVID-19 is not just a viral pandemic; it is also a powerful producer of social isolation for victims of IPV. COVID-19 unlike natural disasters has eliminated children's ability to participate in school and families' ability to practice their religious faith. Victims seeking to attend physician appointments are being redirected to virtual doctor visits, again further socially isolating them from external support systems. There may never have been a more socially isolating event in American history.

Stress

Stress is defined by Cohen et al. (1998) as "environmental demands that tax or exceed the adaptive capacity of an organism, resulting in biological and psychological changes that may be detrimental and place the organism at risk for disease or disability" [6]. Many individuals already suffered from increased overall levels of stress before COVID-19, especially those in minority communities [7]. The Commonwealth Minority Health Survey illustrated racial and ethnic variation in stress. On a global measure combining exposure to stressors in five domains (occupation, finances, relationships, racial bias, and violence), blacks, Hispanics, and Asians reported higher levels of stress than whites [7]. Common stressors have been the following: economic difficulties, physical deprivation, low health status, occupational strain, death of a spouse or loved one, family responsibilities or difficulties, neighborhood instability, and discrimination. COVID-19 not only produces each of these stressors but also can exponentiate their impact in communities. The current pandemic in some ways resembles a natural disaster that is superimposed on current challenges in these communities. Natural disasters are known to produce enormous amounts of stress, and stress hormones are associated with increased aggression [8, 9]. COVID-19 has been demonstrated to be causing high levels of stress both here in America and in communities across the globe [10, 11]. Sequential studies measuring the impact of COVID-19 on stress levels as the pandemic grows and concern for loved ones and economic insecurity escalates have not yet been performed. Investigators at the University of Miami have created the COVID-19 Household Environment Scale which has been developed to measure the impact of the virus on family function, cohesion, and conflict. What simply cannot be understated is the result of the lack of ability to appropriately manage these high stress levels in homes where IPV takes place. While economic insecurity or loss of a job tends to be well-studied initiators of IPV, any adversity experienced within the previous calendar year is associated with an approximately 9% increase in perpetration of IPV by men with childhood challenges [12]. Healthcare providers should anticipate stress overload in their communities and appropriately screen for incidents of IPV particularly when unexplained emergency room visits of irregular injury patterns present themselves.

Substance Abuse

Stress often produces the desire to self-medicate which can lead to overconsumption of addictive substances and impaired judgment. Researchers found that after Hurricane Katrina one third of individuals displaced to Houston, Texas, had increased their consumption of tobacco, alcohol, or marijuana [9]. Similar results can be expected with COVID-19 pandemic. There are well-established associations between substance abuse and IPV [13]. These issues become further complicated because narcotic usage may be compromised due to travel restrictions and closed borders. During the pandemic street supply and potency have been documented as decreased while cost is inflated [14]. Challenges with sustaining habits may lead to added stress and increased IPV. Overconsumption of alcohol leads to a lack of ability to non-violently negotiate conflict and restrain one's self. It also can exacerbate household financial issues. Sales of alcohol products have increased in most states and industry wide are up 27%, and some estimates put online sales of alcohol up 243% during the pandemic [15]. Right alongside alcohol gun sales also skyrocketed with two million guns being sold in March 2020 [16]. Alcohol and gun sales are at their highest during the pandemic creating a truly life threatening environment for victims of IPV.

Economic Insecurity

Job losses in the United States are at 40 million due to the COVID-19 pandemic [17]. Economic insecurity is a well-known stressor leading to increased incidents of IPV [18]. Plans at phased reopening of the economy put in doubt whether older Americans with chronic disease will soon return to work in the same capacity. Most plans call for a tiered return to work prioritizing younger workers who are either recovered from having the virus or are to be tested. Workers who are over the age of 65 and have comorbid conditions that place them in the higher-risk pool have less certain employment futures. And given the likelihood of maintained social distancing practices and a transformed delivery platform for services, many jobs will not return. This perpetual stress is magnified by the fact that victims of IPV may have two very unfortunate outcomes. The first is that they are no longer employed and now have no temporary escape away from the violence. The second is that the abuser is unemployed and now currently is at home continuously. Both of these results are not optimal.

Lack of Accessible Public Resources

A truly regretful event for those suffering from IPV is the lack of accessible public resources during the pandemic. Historically, in many ways in terms of access, it resembled the scale backs seen during human immunodeficiency virus epidemic secondary to public fear. Hospital social workers and visiting consultants for safe haven shelters are clearly a part of the essential work force. The excessive times for clearance for admission to safe haven shelters while awaiting COVID-19 testing results and the consequential elopement of these IPV victims without follow-up or safe discharge are all disappointing and potentially lethal outcomes that have occurred during the pandemic. Children and economic insecurity represent major reasons in which victims return to an abusive home. The inability to appropriately situate children with the victim in a safe haven shelter is predictive of a successful intervention. This requires interfacing with the community closely, and COVID-19 severely diminished these attempts. Hence, recidivism was more likely. Finally, the delay in court proceedings has also been impactful. While restraining orders were still processed, legal services for victims have been seriously impacted. COVID-19 represents a very unfortunate perfect storm for victims of IPV that facilitates their isolation and makes the violence more likely while limiting opportunities for intervention.

According to Centers for Disease Control data, African-American women are most likely to be killed secondary to IPV at a rate of 4.4/100,000 [19]. Unfortunately, we can only expect that these terrible disparities in outcomes will only grow as a result of the pandemic.

Conclusion

COVID-19 represents a socially isolating disease that creates an unfortunate perfect storm for the perpetuation of IPV. It is essential to continue safe haven strategies for victims as well as law enforcement and legal support services that assist in survival.

References

1. UNFPA, with contributions from Avenir Health, Johns Hopkins University (USA) and Victoria University (Australia). April 27, 2020. Impact of the COVID-19 pandemic on family planning and ending gender-based violence, female genital mutilation and child marriage pandemic threatens achievement of the transformative results committed to by UNFPA. UNFPA.
2. Chew L, Ramdas KN. Caught in the storm: the impact of natural disasters on women. New York, NY: The Global Fund for Women; 2005.
3. Lewin T. Shelters Have Empty Beds; Abused Women Stay Home. The New York Times, October 21, 2001, sec. U.S.
4. James SE, Johnson J, Raghavan C. "I couldn't go anywhere": contextualizing violence and drug abuse: a social network study. Violence Against Women. 2004;10:991–1014.
5. Van Wyk JA, Benson MA, Fox GL, DeMaris A. Detangling individual-, partner-, and community-level correlates of partner violence. Crime Delinq. 2003;49:412–38.

6. Cohen S, Kessler R, Gordon L. Measuring stress: a guide for health and social scientists: Oxford University Press; 1998.
7. Williams DR. Race, stress, and mental health: findings from the commonwealth minority health survey. In: Hogue C, Hargraves M, Scott-Collins K, editors. Minority health in America: findings and policy implications from the commonwealth fund minority health survey. Baltimore, MD: Johns Hopkins University Press; 2000. p. 209–43.
8. Bocarino JA, Hoffman SN, Kirchner HL, Erlich PM, Adams RE, et al. Mental health outcomes at the Jersey Shore after Hurricane Sandy. Int J Emerg Mental Health. 2013;15(3):147–58.
9. Cepeda A, Valdez A, Kaplan C, Hill LE. Patterns of substance use among Hurricane Katrina evacuees in Houston, Texas. Disasters. 2010;34(2)
10. American Psychiatric Association. New poll: COVID-19 impacting mental well-being: Americans feeling anxious, especially for loved ones; older adults are less anxious. 25 Mar 2020. Available: https://www.psychiatry.org/newsroom/news-releases/new-poll-covid-19-impacting-mental-well-being-americans-feeling-anxious-especially-for-loved-ones-older-adults-are-less-anxious. Accessed 2 June 2020.
11. Varshney M, Parel JT, Raizada N, Sarin SK. Initial psychological impact of COVID-19 and its correlates in Indian Community: an online (FEEL-COVID) survey. PLoS One. 2020;15(5):e0233874.
12. Roberts AL, McLaughlin KA, Conron KJ, Koenen KC. Adulthood stressors, history of childhood adversity, and risk of perpetration of intimate partner violence. Am J Prev Med. 2011;40(2):128–38.
13. Karakurt G, Koç E, Çetinsaya EE, Ayluçtarhan Z, Bolen S. Meta-analysis and systematic review for the treatment of perpetrators of intimate partner violence. Neurosci Biobehav Rev. 2019;105:220–30.
14. UN News. May 7, 2020. COVID-19 causes some illegal drug prices to surge, as supplies are disrupted worldwide. https://news.un.org/en/story/2020/05/1063512. Accessed on June 20, 2020.
15. Sweeney D. June 10, 2020. Alcohol sales surge during pandemic, lockdowns. Here's what people are drinking. https://www.miamiherald.com/news/coronavirus/article243433136.html. Accessed on 20 June 2020.
16. Collins K, Yaffey B. D. April 2, 2020. About 2 million guns were sold in the U.S. as virus fears spread. New York Times https://www.nytimes.com/interactive/2020/04/01/business/coronavirus-gun-sales.html. Accessed on 20 June 2020.
17. Aratani L. May 28, 2020. US job losses pass 40m as coronavirus crisis sees claims rise 2.1m in a week. The Guardian https://www.theguardian.com/business/2020/may/28/us-job-losses-unemployment-coronavirus. Accessed on 20 June 2020.
18. Schwab-Reese LM, Peek-Asa C, Parker E. Associations of financial stressors and physical intimate partner violence perpetration. Epidemiology. 2016;3(1):6. Published online 2016 Mar 1.
19. Petrosky E, Blair JM, Betz CJ, Fowler KA, Jack SP, Lyons BH. Racial and ethnic differences in homicides of adult women and the role of intimate partner violence — United States, 2003–2014. MMWR Morb Mortal Wkly Rep. 2017;66:741–6.

Appendix

Dr. Bailey has taken on the issue of Violence from various perspectives. However, the issue of Intimate Partner Violence is in many ways the most challenging and most painful. This book may be Dr. Bailey's most important contribution.

–David Sacher M.D., P.h.D.
16th Surgeon General of the
United States and former Secretary for Health
in the Department of Health and Human Services.

R. K. Bailey (ed.), *Intimate Partner Violence*,
https://doi.org/10.1007/978-3-030-55864-2

Index

R. K. Bailey (ed.), *Intimate Partner Violence*,
https://doi.org/10.1007/978-3-030-55864-2

I

L

M

MIX
Papier aus verantwortungsvollen Quellen
Paper from responsible sources
FSC® C105338

If you have any concerns about our products,
you can contact us on
ProductSafety@springernature.com

In case Publisher is established outside the EU,
the EU authorized representative is:
Springer Nature Customer Service Center GmbH
Europaplatz 3, 69115 Heidelberg, Germany

Printed by Libri Plureos GmbH
in Hamburg, Germany